CARNIVORE COOKBOOK ON A BUDGET

Affordable Meat-Based Recipes for Everyday Health and Simplicity

Emerald Wren Maddox

GRAPEVINE BOOKS

Published by
GRAPEVINE BOOKS

www.grapevinebooks.com
email: contact@grapevinebooks.com

Ordering Information:
Quantity sales: Special discounts are available on quantity purchases by corporations, associations, and others.
For details, reach out to the publisher.

First published by Grapevine Books, 2025

Contents

PART 1

Understanding the Carnivore Diet

PART 2

Essential Techniques

PART 3

Core Recipes

PART 1

Understanding the Carnivore Diet

Origins, Principles, and Why Everyone's Talking About It

If you've ever wished you could just eat steak and bacon all day and still feel like you're doing something good for your body—welcome to the Carnivore Diet. It sounds extreme at first (no plants at all?), but the idea is surprisingly simple: eat only animal-based foods and eliminate everything else. That means meat, fish, eggs, and animal fats—no veggies, no fruits, no grains, and definitely no sugar.

So, Where Did This Come From?

Believe it or not, this isn't some TikTok trend that blew up last week. The roots of the carnivore diet stretch back centuries, if not millennia. Just look at traditional societies like the Inuit in the Arctic or the Maasai in Africa. These cultures thrived on meat-heavy or even meat-only diets, often with no signs of modern diseases like diabetes or heart issues.

Fast forward to the modern world, and the carnivore movement has been spearheaded by people like Dr. Shawn Baker (a former orthopedic surgeon and weightlifting beast) and Mikhaila Peterson (who swears by it for managing autoimmune conditions). With the rise of podcasts, Instagram influencers, and #meatheals hashtags, the diet has exploded in popularity among people frustrated by food sensitivities, digestive issues, or the endless noise of conflicting nutrition advice.

You're not alone if you've felt overwhelmed by trying to "eat healthy" and still felt bloated, tired, or just plain confused. The carnivore diet offers a bold reset button. Strip away the noise, simplify your plate, and see how your body reacts.

What's the Point of Cutting Out Plants?

Here's where things get spicy. While we've all been told that kale and broccoli are health foods, carnivore enthusiasts argue that many plants actually contain natural defense chemicals—like oxalates and lectins—that can irritate your gut, trigger inflammation, and mess with your immune system.

The thinking is this: your body doesn't *need* carbs or fiber to function. It can run beautifully on fat and protein. When you eliminate all plant-based foods, you're removing common allergens, anti-nutrients, and sugar spikes. What you're left with is a diet that's incredibly nutrient-dense, easy to digest, and surprisingly satisfying. No calorie counting. No "What am I allowed to eat today?" headaches. Just real food, eaten when you're hungry, until you're full.

The Basic Rules (Don't Worry—They're Simple)

Ready? Here's what you *can* eat:

- Beef, pork, lamb, chicken, turkey, bison, elk—basically all meats
- Fatty fish like salmon, sardines, and mackerel
- Eggs (especially yolks)
- Animal fats: butter, tallow, suet
- Bone broth
- Salt, water, and maybe black coffee if you're not going hardcore

That's it. No grains. No beans. No fruit smoothies. And definitely no oat milk lattes.

Sound restrictive? Maybe. But for many people, it's *liberating*. You always know what's on the menu, your grocery list is shorter, and you stop obsessing over food choices. Plus, steak tastes better than salad anyway.

Carnivore vs Keto vs Paleo vs Primal: What's the Difference?

Let's break it down.

- **Keto** is low-carb and high-fat, but it still includes some plant foods like leafy greens, nuts, and avocado. It's focused on staying in ketosis (burning fat instead of carbs), and you'll often track macros. Carnivore skips the math and just says: eat meat.
- **Paleo** is about eating like a caveman—meat, veggies, fruits, nuts, seeds—but it avoids dairy, grains, and processed foods. It's clean eating, but still plant-heavy.
- **Primal** is like paleo's laid-back cousin. It includes everything paleo does but allows for some raw dairy and modern foods, like dark chocolate or fermented goods. It's flexible, but not meat-exclusive.
- **Carnivore**? That's the minimalist version. Meat only. It's the ultimate elimination diet, the reset your body didn't know it needed. You don't worry about ketone levels or caveman logic. You just eat like a lion.

Why Is This Diet So Popular Now?

Three words: results, simplicity, and rebellion. People are seeing huge transformations—weight loss, clearer skin, better energy, improved digestion—by eating what nutritionists once told us would clog our arteries. The carnivore diet flips mainstream nutrition on its head, and people love that.

It's also insanely simple. No barcodes to scan. No 20-ingredient "superfood" salads. No complicated recipes. Just cook some meat, salt it, and enjoy.

And let's be honest—there's something fun about being a little rebellious with your diet. When everyone else is sipping green juice, you're biting into a ribeye. When they're debating almond milk vs oat milk, you're pouring bacon grease over your eggs.

In the end, the carnivore diet isn't about being extreme for the sake of it. It's about getting back to basics, listening to your body, and fueling yourself with foods we've been eating for thousands of years. And if you love meat? Well, you're going to feel right at home.

Health Benefits & Risks of the Carnivore Diet

So, you're intrigued by the idea of eating nothing but meat. Maybe you've heard the stories—people dropping pounds, clearing up lifelong gut issues, finally feeling energized after years of chronic fatigue. Sounds great, right? But before you dive headfirst into a plate of ribeyes, let's take a closer look at what the carnivore diet can do for your body—and what you should keep in mind along the way.

The Good Stuff: Health Benefits

1. Gut Health: Goodbye Bloat, Hello Simplicity

If your stomach has ever turned into a bloated balloon after a "healthy" meal of salad, quinoa, and beans, you're not alone. One of the biggest draws of the carnivore diet is its gut-calming effect.

By cutting out all fiber-rich and plant-based foods, you're eliminating common irritants like lectins, oxalates, and FODMAPs—things that can cause gas, bloating, or even pain for sensitive individuals. Many people with IBS, Crohn's, or chronic digestive issues find relief on carnivore simply because there's less to trigger a reaction.

It's basically the ultimate elimination diet. Meat is one of the least reactive foods you can eat. That's why so many people who've spent years juggling food intolerances say their digestion becomes smooth, quiet, and stress-free after switching to carnivore.

2. Weight Loss: Meat, Fat, and a Shrinking Waistline

Here's the wild part: most people on the carnivore diet eat until they're full—no calorie counting, no portion control—and still lose weight. How?

For one, meat is incredibly satiating. You're getting protein and fat, which naturally reduce hunger hormones and keep blood sugar stable. That means fewer cravings, less snacking, and no energy crashes.

Plus, without carbs spiking insulin levels, your body becomes a fat-burning machine. Many carnivore dieters enter a state of mild ketosis (burning fat for energy instead of carbs) without even trying.

Also, no more "sneaky" calories from sauces, snacks, and sugar-filled extras. When your meals are meat-based, you're eating clean by default.

3. Energy Levels: From Sluggish to Supercharged

Let's be real: when you're eating a standard Western diet full of sugar and processed food, your energy levels are all over the place. You crash mid-afternoon. You feel foggy by 7 p.m. You need coffee to function.

Carnivore often flips that switch. Without blood sugar spikes and dips, your energy becomes steady and reliable. Some people even report needing less sleep, feeling sharper mentally, and waking up without an alarm for the first time in years.

This happens because fat is a more efficient fuel for the brain, and once your body adapts to burning it full-time, you may notice improved mental clarity, better mood, and fewer slumps.

The Other Side: Risks & Concerns

Of course, the carnivore diet isn't without its critics. You've probably heard warnings like "But what about fiber?" or "Isn't all that red meat bad for your heart?" Let's walk through some of the most common concerns—and what the science (and real-life experience) says.

1. Nutrients: Are You Missing Out?

One big worry is nutrient deficiency. No fruits? No veggies? Surely you'll be missing key vitamins and minerals, right?

Surprisingly, meat is more nutrient-dense than most people think. Red meat provides:

- **Iron** (in its most absorbable form, heme iron)
- **B vitamins**, including B12
- **Zinc, selenium, and phosphorus**
- **Fat-soluble vitamins** like A, D, E, and K (especially in organ meats)

Organ meats like liver are basically nature's multivitamin. If you incorporate nose-to-tail eating—like liver, heart, marrow, and eggs—you can cover almost every essential nutrient.

Still, some people supplement with magnesium or electrolytes, especially during the first few weeks as their bodies adapt. It's all about listening to how *your* body responds.

2. Cholesterol and Heart Health: Is Red Meat Dangerous?

This is the big one. The conventional wisdom says saturated fat and cholesterol raise your risk of heart disease. But the science has been shifting.

Recent studies show that dietary cholesterol doesn't necessarily raise blood cholesterol in most people. And when you're not combining meat with processed carbs, seed oils, or sugar, the inflammatory effects are much lower.

Many people on carnivore actually see improved blood markers: lower triglycerides, higher HDL ("good" cholesterol), and reduced inflammation. LDL might go up—but context matters. The pattern of LDL (small dense vs large buoyant) is a better predictor of heart risk than total numbers.

If you have a history of heart disease or concerns about cholesterol, it's wise to track your labs, work with a functional or open-minded doctor, and focus on high-quality, unprocessed animal foods.

3. Fiber: Don't You Need It to Poop?

Short answer: not necessarily.

It might sound weird, but many people on carnivore have regular (if less frequent) bowel movements despite eating zero fiber. Why? Because when your gut isn't inflamed and your body is efficiently absorbing nutrients, there's less waste to eliminate.

Fiber can help *some* people with constipation, but for others—especially those with IBS or gut sensitivity—it can actually make things worse.

Still, your poop schedule might change on carnivore. That's normal. As long as you're not in pain or excessively backed up, your body's likely just adjusting.

The Bottom Line

Every diet has trade-offs. The carnivore diet isn't magic—but for many people, it's powerful. It strips away the clutter, focuses on nutrient-dense, bioavailable food, and removes common triggers that could be wrecking your health without you even realizing it.

You don't need to go all-in forever. Some people try it for 30 days to reset their system, then add back other foods slowly. Others stay full carnivore and thrive. The key is to experiment, stay curious, and let *your* body be the final judge.

Because in the end, the best diet is the one that actually makes you feel good—and keeps you there.

What You Can and Can't Eat on the Carnivore Diet

One of the best parts of the carnivore diet is how *easy* it is to follow. No macros, no calorie tracking, no endless ingredient lists. It's straightforward: eat animal-based foods and skip everything else. Still, if you're new to this way of eating, you might wonder about the gray areas. Is coffee okay? What about dairy? Bacon? Let's clear that up.

At its core, the carnivore diet focuses on animal foods: meat, eggs, and fat. That's your "yes" list. Then there's the "no" list—plants, sugar, grains, and processed junk. But in between, there's a "maybe" zone—foods that some carnivores include based on personal preference or goals.

This table gives you a quick visual breakdown:

✔ What's In, ✘ What's Out, and 🤔 What's Up to You

YES – Eat Freely	Maybe / Use Sparingly	NO / Eliminate Completely
Beef, lamb, pork, bison	Coffee / tea (unsweetened)	Vegetables (broccoli, spinach, kale etc.)
Chicken, turkey, duck	Hard cheeses / full-fat dairy	Fruits and fruit juice
Organ meats (liver, kidney, heart)	Heavy cream	Grains (wheat, oats, rice, etc.)
Fish (salmon, sardines, mackerel)	Butter / ghee	Legumes (beans, lentils, soy)
Eggs (any style)	Bacon (watch ingredients)	Seed oils (canola, soybean, sunflower)
Animal fats (tallow, lard, suet)	Seasonings (no additives)	Sugar and sweeteners (natural or fake)
Salt (sea salt, Redmond, Himalayan)	Sparkling water / mineral water	Packaged snacks, protein bars
Bone broth	Supplements (if needed)	Alcohol, soda, juices
Shellfish	Raw milk (for primal types)	Nuts and seeds

Let's Break It Down

☑ What You *Can* Eat Freely

This is your core: meat, eggs, and fat. Whether it's a ribeye, sardines, scrambled eggs, or a slab of liver, these foods are nutrient-dense, satisfying, and totally carnivore-approved. Fat is your fuel source here, so don't skimp on it—tallow, butter, and egg yolks are your friends.

❌ What You *Shouldn't* Eat

Plants and processed foods are out. No kale chips, quinoa, apples, or almond butter. The idea is to eliminate foods that cause inflammation, gut issues, or blood sugar spikes. Even "healthy" options like oatmeal or smoothies don't belong here—they're full of sugar or anti-nutrients.

🤔 What's in the Gray Area

Some carnivores include coffee, dairy, or spices, while others go strict and cut out everything but meat, fat, and salt. You'll see terms like "Lion Diet" (super strict: only ruminant meat, salt, water) and "relaxed carnivore" (includes coffee, butter, cream, etc.). Find what works for *you*, especially in the beginning. Just aim for simplicity and minimal processing.

If you're ever unsure about a food, just ask yourself:

Did it once have a face? Or come from something that did?

If yes—chances are, it's carnivore-approved.

PART 2

Essential Techniques

Tools & Pantry Staples

Starting the carnivore diet isn't just about changing what you eat—it's about changing how you *cook* and shop. You're going to be preparing a lot of meat, eggs, and fat, so having the right tools makes the process smoother, faster, and more enjoyable. Whether you're a seasoned home cook or someone who barely knows how to turn on the stove, this guide will give you everything you need to feel confident in your carnivore kitchen.

🔪 Must-Have Cooking Tools for Carnivore Success

You don't need a fancy chef's kitchen to thrive on carnivore—but investing in a few solid tools will make your life much easier. These are the game-changers:

1. Cast Iron Skillet

This is your go-to for searing steaks, crisping pork belly, frying eggs, or even roasting a whole chicken thigh-side down. Cast iron gets screaming hot, holds heat like a champ, and develops an amazing crust on your meat. Bonus: it lasts a lifetime.

2. Meat Thermometer

When you're cooking meat every day, you want it *just right*. A digital thermometer helps you nail doneness without guesswork. No more cutting open your ribeye and hoping it's not overcooked.

3. Air Fryer or Oven

Want crispy bacon or tender chicken thighs without splatter? An air fryer is a carnivore's secret weapon. It gives you that golden crust with minimal cleanup. A conventional oven works just as well—just grab a wire rack for better airflow.

4. Slow Cooker or Instant Pot

Perfect for tougher cuts like brisket, oxtail, pork shoulder, or beef cheeks. These tools turn collagen-rich cuts into tender, fall-apart magic with almost zero effort. Set it, forget it, feast.

5. Cutting Boards & Sharp Knives

If you're prepping meat often, invest in a large cutting board (preferably wood or BPA-free plastic) and a solid chef's knife or boning knife. Sharp knives make trimming fat or slicing liver much more pleasant (and safer).

6. Blender or Food Processor (Optional)

For those who like making organ meat blends, egg-based sauces, or even meat-only "pâtés," a small processor or stick blender comes in handy.

7. Glass Storage Containers or Meal Prep Trays

You'll likely cook in batches—especially with roasts or broths. Glass containers help you store meat safely, reheat evenly, and keep your fridge organized.

🛒 Your Carnivore Shopping List

Think of your pantry and fridge as your personal meat vault. Stocking up on the right cuts and fats makes it easier to stay on track and mix things up. Here's a breakdown of what to have on hand:

🥩 Meat (The Star of the Show)

Red Meat – the core of most carnivore diets:

- Ribeye (fatty, flavorful, indulgent)
- Ground beef (80/20 for ideal fat-protein balance)
- Chuck roast (great for slow cooking)
- Brisket (tender and collagen-rich)
- Short ribs
- Steak cuts: NY Strip, sirloin, filet mignon
- Oxtail, beef cheeks (great for stews)

- Lamb chops or shoulder
- Pork belly, pork chops, ham hocks
- Ground lamb or pork

Poultry:

- Chicken thighs (skin-on, bone-in for best flavor)
- Whole chicken (roast it, then use the bones for broth)
- Turkey legs or ground turkey
- Duck breasts (for crispy skin lovers)

Game Meats (optional):

- Venison
- Elk
- Bison
- Wild boar

🥚 Eggs & Dairy (Optional for Most)

- Eggs (get a few dozen—you'll use them daily)
- Heavy cream (if tolerated)
- Butter (grass-fed like Kerrygold, if possible)
- Ghee or clarified butter
- Hard cheeses (parmesan, cheddar—go easy if sensitive)

Organ Meats (Nature's Multivitamin)

These are nutrient-dense powerhouses. Even a small amount once or twice a week can make a huge difference:

- Beef liver (start slow—it's potent)
- Chicken liver (milder taste)
- Heart (beef or chicken—chewy, but delicious when cooked right)
- Kidneys (can be sautéed in butter)
- Spleen, thymus (advanced level!)
- Bone marrow (roast and eat by the spoonful)

If the idea of organs freaks you out, try blending liver into ground beef at a 90:10 ratio. You won't taste it, but you'll still get the benefits.

Animal Fats & Oils

- Tallow (rendered beef fat—great for frying or roasting)
- Lard (rendered pork fat—perfect for eggs and pan-frying)
- Suet (raw beef fat—can be rendered at home)
- Duck fat (insanely flavorful for searing)
- Bone marrow (spoon it on steaks, mix into ground beef)
- Butter or ghee (if tolerated—some prefer dairy-free)

These fats are essential on carnivore. They're your energy source, and they make meat taste amazing. You want to *embrace* the fat, not fear it.

🧂 Spices, Salts & Add-Ons

The strictest carnivores use only salt and water. But many include a few extras for flavor:

- Salt (Redmond Real Salt, Himalayan pink salt, sea salt)
- Pepper (optional—some eliminate it)
- Garlic powder, onion powder (mild irritants for some)
- Dried herbs like rosemary or thyme (optional)
- Apple cider vinegar (a few drops for tenderizing meats)
- Mustard (if not sensitive—check for additives)
- Bone broth (homemade or clean store-bought)

🧊 Bonus: Stocking the Freezer

Buying in bulk saves money. If you've got freezer space, consider grabbing:

- 10-lb briskets or pork shoulders
- Ground meat in 5-lb packs
- Organ meat blends
- Marrow bones for roasting
- Large bones for broth batches

Pro tip: pre-portion your meat into 1-lb or meal-sized packs before freezing, so you're always ready to grab, thaw, and cook.

🧼 Keep It Simple, Keep It Clean

Once your pantry is stocked and your tools are set, carnivore cooking becomes effortless. No need to overthink meals, prep sauces, or juggle sides. Your entire kitchen revolves around one question: *What meat do I want today, and how do I want to cook it?*

So go ahead—fire up that skillet, throw some tallow in the pan, and sear yourself a steak. With the right gear and staples, you're already halfway to carnivore mastery.

How to Cook Meat Right

If meat is the star of your diet, then cooking it well is your superpower. You don't need to be a professional chef or own fancy kitchen gear to make your meals taste incredible—you just need a few techniques that bring out the flavor, texture, and juiciness in every cut. Whether you're searing steaks on the stovetop, slow-roasting a brisket, or tossing bacon in the air fryer, knowing how to cook meat *right* can make the carnivore lifestyle feel like a daily feast.

🔥 1. Grilling: That Flame-Kissed Magic

Grilling is primal—and delicious. Few things compare to the smoky flavor of meat kissed by an open flame. It's perfect for steaks, ribs, burgers, chicken thighs, and sausages.

Tips for Better Grilling:

- **Let your meat sit at room temperature** for 20–30 minutes before grilling. Cold meat won't cook evenly.
- **Preheat the grill properly.** For gas, crank it up and close the lid to get those grates screaming hot. For charcoal, wait until the coals are glowing white.
- **Use tallow or beef fat** to oil the grates. This prevents sticking and adds flavor.
- **Don't press your meat.** You're not trying to drain the juice—let it stay in!
- **Rest after grilling.** Let your meat sit for 5–10 minutes so the juices redistribute.

Grilling is ideal for fattier cuts like ribeye, pork chops, and lamb, where that high heat creates a crust while the inside stays tender.

🍳 2. Pan-Frying: Crispy, Juicy, and Fast

Pan-frying gives you total control. It's fast, easy, and perfect for everyday meals. Whether it's searing a steak or crisping up chicken thighs, pan-frying delivers serious flavor thanks to the Maillard reaction—that golden-brown crust that makes meat irresistible.

Key Techniques:

- **Use a heavy skillet.** Cast iron or stainless steel holds heat best.

- **Get your pan hot first.** Then add fat—tallow, lard, or ghee are best. Wait until it shimmers before adding meat.

- **Avoid crowding.** Overcrowding traps steam, and instead of browning, you'll be boiling.

- **Sear, then lower heat.** Start with a high-heat sear to form the crust, then reduce the heat to finish cooking through.

- **Deglaze if you want extra flavor.** After cooking, you can add a splash of bone broth to loosen the fond (browned bits) for a rich sauce.

This method is great for steaks, pork belly slices, burgers, liver, and eggs. It's especially handy when you want that golden crisp outside with a tender middle—without firing up a grill.

🐢 3. Slow-Cooking: Low and Slow for Maximum Tenderness

When it comes to tough cuts like brisket, oxtail, short ribs, or beef cheeks, low and slow is the name of the game. These cuts are full of connective tissue that breaks down during long cooking, turning into rich, melt-in-your-mouth bites.

Slow-Cooking Essentials:

- **Use moisture.** Add some bone broth, beef fat, or water to the bottom of the pot. It helps break down collagen.

- **Season simply.** Salt is all you need. You can add pepper, garlic, or herbs if you're flexible.

- **Set it and forget it.** Use a crockpot or Dutch oven and let it go for 6–8 hours on low.

- **Shred and store.** Slow-cooked meats are perfect for batch cooking. Shred them, add fat to keep them moist, and store in glass containers for quick meals all week.

This method is unbeatable for meal prep and perfect for those days when you don't want to hover over a stove. Bonus: your house will smell amazing.

4. Air-Frying: Crispy Without the Mess

Air fryers have become a favorite in the carnivore community—and for good reason. They give you crisp edges, juicy centers, and super quick cook times without splatter or smoke.

Best Practices:

- **Don't overload the basket.** Leave space so the hot air can circulate.
- **Flip halfway.** Especially for bacon or burgers, flipping gives you even crisping.
- **Use parchment paper sparingly.** It's okay, but don't cover everything—airflow is key.
- **Watch cook times.** Air fryers run hot. A 1-inch pork chop might be done in 8–10 minutes. Burgers take 6–7. Chicken wings? Around 20.

Great for crispy chicken thighs, meatballs, sausages, burger patties, bacon, or even reheating leftovers without drying them out.

Final Tips for Perfect Meat Every Time

- **Salt before or after—but not too early.** Salting meat 5–10 minutes before cooking is ideal. Too early, and it pulls out moisture.
- **Let meat rest after cooking.** This locks in juices and keeps everything tender.
- **Don't fear fat.** The tastiest meat is often the fattier cut—embrace it!
- **Use a meat thermometer.** Seriously. It's the difference between dry and dreamy.

Whether you're grilling on the patio, frying eggs in tallow, or slow-cooking a giant roast while working from home, these methods will help you get the best out of every cut of meat. Cooking carnivore doesn't have to be complicated—but it should always be delicious.

Fat Management

Fat isn't just allowed on the carnivore diet—it's essential. When you're running on animal foods, fat becomes your primary fuel source. It keeps you full, fuels your brain, and supports hormone health. But managing fat well—both in cooking and eating—makes all the difference in how you feel and how satisfying your meals are.

🔥 Cooking Fats: What to Use and When

- **Tallow** (rendered beef fat) is perfect for high-heat cooking like searing steaks or pan-frying burgers. It has a neutral flavor and a high smoke point.
- **Butter** adds richness and flavor but contains small amounts of dairy solids. If you're sensitive to dairy, use **ghee**—clarified butter with milk solids removed.
- **Lard** (rendered pork fat) is great for eggs, pork chops, or baking-style carnivore recipes.
- **Duck fat** is luxurious and flavorful—great for special meals or crispy chicken skin.

🧈 Suet & Rendering Your Own Fat

Suet is raw beef or lamb fat, especially from around the kidneys. It's firm and dry, ideal for rendering into tallow. To render:

1. Chop suet into small pieces.
2. Simmer on low in a heavy pot or slow cooker until melted.
3. Strain through cheesecloth into a glass jar.
4. Let cool and store refrigerated.

Rendered fat stores well and can be used for cooking or drizzled over lean meats for extra satiety.

🧂 Fat as Fuel

Aim for fatty cuts like ribeye, pork belly, and 80/20 ground beef. If your meat is too lean, add tallow or butter on top. Balance is key—too little fat, and you'll feel sluggish or hungry; too much too soon, and digestion may protest.

Start simple, listen to your body, and embrace the fat.

Eggs, Bone Broth, and More

Steak might be the superstar of the carnivore diet, but it's far from the only tool in your toolbox. If you're eating animal-based long-term, variety matters—not just for flavor, but for nutrients, texture, and digestion. Thankfully, there's a world of simple, nourishing options beyond your daily ribeye. Eggs, bone broth, and lesser-known staples can round out your diet and elevate your carnivore experience without requiring complicated prep.

🥚 Eggs: The Unsung Hero of Simplicity

Eggs are a carnivore staple for a reason. They're quick to cook, easy to digest, and packed with nutrition. A single egg contains protein, fat, choline, selenium, B vitamins, and even small amounts of vitamin D and iron—all wrapped in one tiny shell.

Best Ways to Eat Them:

- **Scrambled in butter or tallow** for a fluffy, rich breakfast
- **Boiled or poached** as a quick snack or side
- **Fried in bacon fat or ghee** for a crispy edge
- **Omelet-style with leftover ground meat or shredded roast**

If you're sensitive to egg whites, you can stick to just the yolks, which contain most of the nutrients anyway. For most people, though, whole eggs are well tolerated and incredibly versatile.

Pro tip: Add a yolk to freshly cooked ground beef or liver. It boosts fat and creaminess, turning a basic dish into a rich, silky treat.

🍲 Bone Broth: Carnivore Gold in a Mug

Bone broth is the warm hug your gut didn't know it needed. It's made by simmering bones, marrow, joints, and connective tissue for hours to extract collagen, gelatin, amino acids, and minerals. While it's not essential, it's a fantastic addition—especially during the adaptation phase or when recovering from illness.

Benefits of Bone Broth:

- Soothes digestion and heals the gut lining

- Supports joints and skin thanks to collagen and glycine
- Replenishes electrolytes like sodium, potassium, and magnesium
- Helps with hydration, especially when you're skipping carbs and fiber

How to Make It:

1. Use leftover bones (beef, lamb, chicken, etc.).
2. Add water to cover and a dash of salt.
3. Simmer on low for 12–24 hours.
4. Strain, cool, and store in glass jars.

Drink it as a warm beverage, or use it to cook tougher cuts of meat. It can also be poured over meals as a rich "gravy" alternative.

🫀 Don't Forget the Off-Cuts: Fat, Marrow & Organs

Carnivore isn't just about muscle meat. The more you eat *nose-to-tail*, the more well-rounded your nutrition becomes. If steak is the foundation, these extras are the bricks that make the house solid.

- • **Bone Marrow:** Roast marrow bones at 450°F for 15–20 minutes until soft. Scoop out and spread over meat or mix into ground beef for an instant fat boost.
- • **Rendered Fats (like tallow or lard):** Cook lean cuts like sirloin or chicken breast in extra fat for satiety.
- • **Organs (like liver, heart, kidney):** Even small amounts once a week provide massive micronutrient benefits. Blend into ground meat or sauté in butter with salt.

🧈 Fat Bombs, Egg-Based Sides & Carnivore Hacks

Looking to get more fat in without feeling stuffed? Here are a few clever additions:

- **Hard-boiled eggs with butter or salt**

- **Egg yolk "butter"** (soft yolks blended with ghee or tallow)
- **Beef fat bites**: rendered tallow cooled into cubes and seasoned lightly with salt

While these aren't required daily, they help if you're struggling with hunger, energy dips, or are on leaner cuts of meat.

💡 Keeping It Interesting

Carnivore doesn't have to mean boring. When you incorporate eggs, broths, off-cuts, and fats into your weekly routine, you open up tons of variety without compromising your goals. A sample day might look like:

- **Breakfast:** Scrambled eggs in bacon grease with leftover brisket
- **Lunch:** Ground beef topped with melted marrow and sea salt
- **Dinner:** Slow-cooked short ribs in bone broth
- **Bonus:** A mug of broth before bed, or a boiled egg with butter for a quick snack

These staples make your meals satisfying, balanced, and deeply nourishing—without needing a single plant-based ingredient.

In short, while steak is great, carnivore living thrives on variety. Eggs, bone broth, and fat-rich extras help fill nutritional gaps, support digestion, and keep your meals exciting without breaking the rules. Think of them not as add-ons, but as essential elements of a powerful, sustainable way of eating.

PART 3

Core Recipes

Pot Roast

Here's a simple, hearty **Carnivore-Style Pot Roast** recipe—no veggies, no carbs, just rich, tender meat with collagen-rich broth and satisfying fat.

Carnivore Pot Roast
Yield: 4 to 6 servings
Prep Time: 10 minutes
Cook Time: 3 to 4 hours

Ingredients:

- 3 to 4 lb **chuck roast** (or brisket)
- 2 tbsp **beef tallow** (or lard/butter)
- 2 tsp **sea salt** (adjust to taste)
- 2 cups **bone broth** (beef or lamb)
- Optional: 1 tsp **garlic powder** or black pepper (for non-strict carnivore)

Instructions:

1. Sear the Meat

In a large Dutch oven or heavy-bottomed pot, heat tallow over medium-high heat. Pat the roast dry with paper towels, season with salt, and sear it on all sides until deeply browned (about 3–4 minutes per side). This helps lock in flavor.

2. Deglaze with Broth

Once seared, pour in the bone broth to deglaze the pot, scraping up any browned bits from the bottom. These add rich, meaty flavor.

3. Slow Cook

Cover with a lid and reduce the heat to low. Let the roast simmer for 3 to 4 hours, checking occasionally to ensure it stays partially submerged. Flip halfway through for even cooking.

4. Shred & Serve

Once fork-tender, shred the roast with two forks or slice thickly. Serve with a spoonful of the fatty broth poured over top.

Tips:

- For extra fat, add a few marrow bones to the pot during cooking.
- Store leftovers in broth to keep them moist and flavorful.

> Perfect for batch cooking or sharing—this pot roast is a carnivore comfort classic.

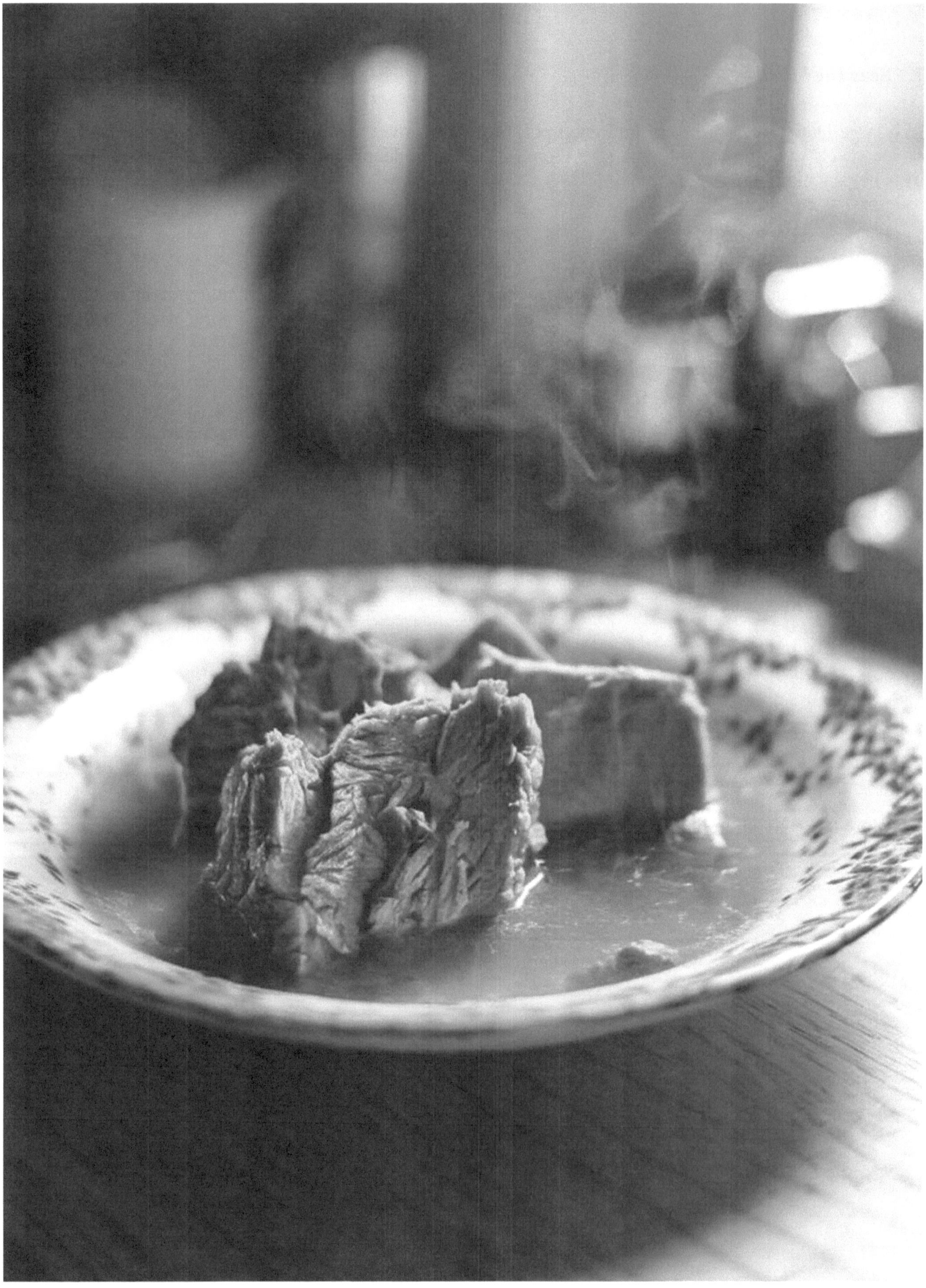

Pot Smoked-Style Brisket

Here's a tender, juicy **Instant Pot Smoked-Style Brisket** recipe designed for carnivore dieters—rich, flavorful, and done in a fraction of the time. While you won't get the classic smoke ring from a smoker, this version uses seasoning and technique to mimic the deep flavor of slow-smoked meat using your Instant Pot.

Instant Pot Smoked Brisket

Yield: 6 servings

Prep Time: 10 minutes

Cook Time: 90 minutes + natural release

Total Time: ~2 hours

Ingredients:

- 2.5 to 3 lb **brisket flat or point cut**
- 1 tbsp **tallow or butter**
- 2 tsp **sea salt**
- 1 tsp **smoked salt** *(optional, for smoke flavor)*
- 1 tsp **garlic powder** *(optional, omit for strict carnivore)*
- 1 cup **bone broth** or water

Instructions:

1. Season the Brisket

Pat the brisket dry with paper towels. Rub all sides with sea salt and smoked salt. For added flavor, sprinkle with garlic powder if using.

2. Sear the Brisket (Optional but recommended)

Set the Instant Pot to *Sauté*. Add tallow or butter and sear the brisket for 3–4 minutes per side until browned. This adds depth and a crust-like texture.

3. Deglaze and Pressure Cook

Remove the brisket. Add bone broth to deglaze the pot, scraping up browned bits. Return the brisket, fatty side up. Seal the lid.

4. Pressure Cook

Set to *Manual/High Pressure* for **90 minutes**. Let pressure release naturally for 20 minutes, then do a quick release if needed.

5. Rest & Slice

Transfer the brisket to a board. Let rest 10–15 minutes. Slice against the grain or shred, spooning juices over the top.

Tips:

- For a smoky crust, sear again in a skillet or under a broiler for 5–10 minutes after pressure cooking.
- Save the cooking juices! They're rich in flavor and perfect for reheating or drizzling over servings.

> This method delivers smoky, fall-apart brisket with minimal fuss—and it's 100% carnivore compliant.

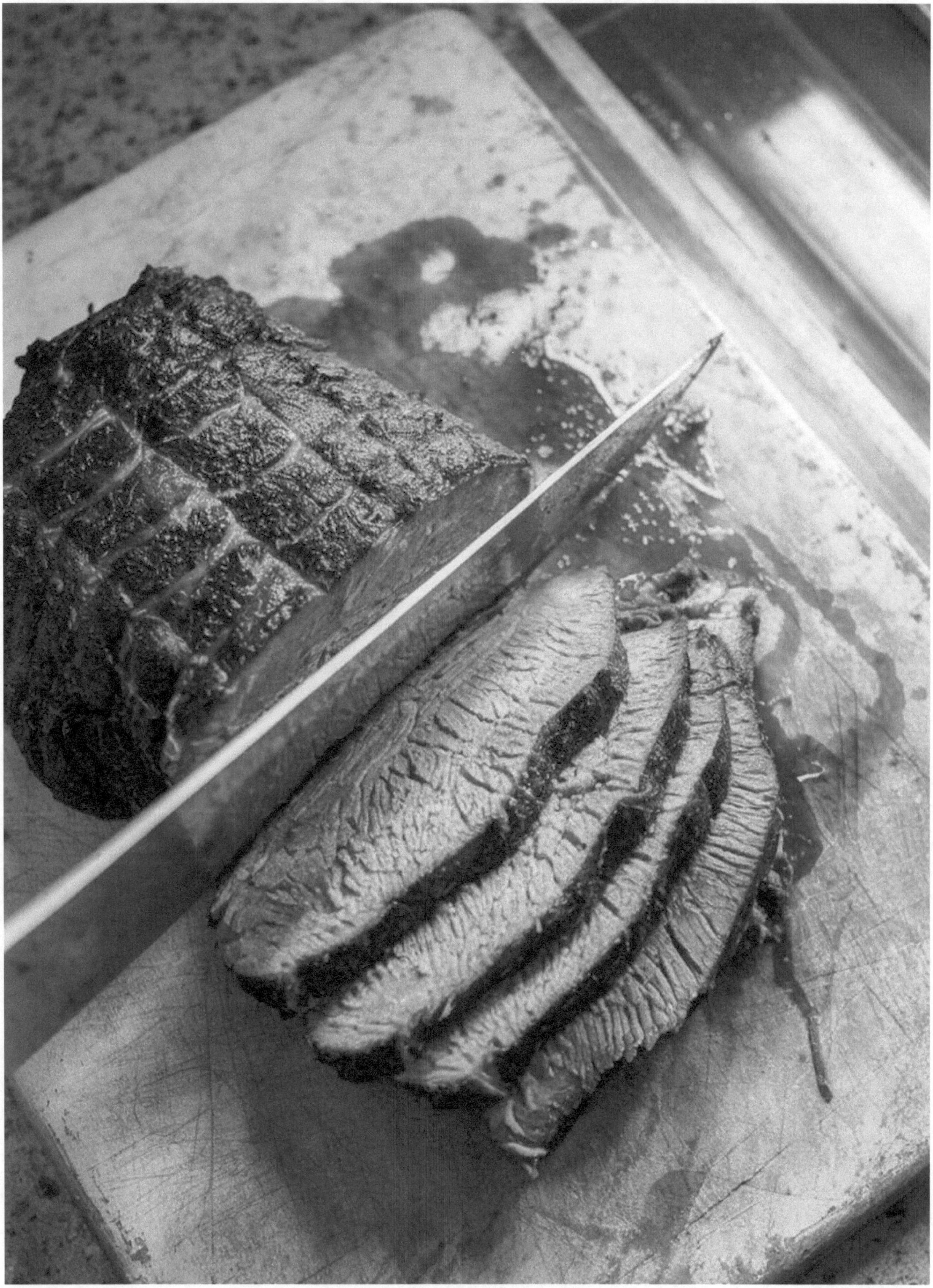

Crispy Chicken Thighs

Here's a foolproof recipe for **Crispy Chicken Thighs**—carnivore-style. These are juicy on the inside with golden, crackly skin on the outside, using minimal ingredients and maximum flavor.

Crispy Chicken Thighs
Yield: 4 servings
Prep Time: 5 minutes
Cook Time: 25–30 minutes
Total Time: ~35 minutes

Ingredients:

- 4 **bone-in, skin-on chicken thighs**
- 1 tsp **sea salt**
- 1 tbsp **beef tallow**, duck fat, or butter
- Optional: ½ tsp **garlic powder** or **black pepper** (omit for strict carnivore)

Instructions (Stovetop + Oven Method):

1. **Preheat Oven**

Preheat your oven to **425°F (220°C)**.

2. **Season the Thighs**

Pat chicken thighs dry with paper towels (very important for crispiness). Season skin and underside with salt.

3. **Sear Skin-Side Down**

Heat a cast iron or oven-safe skillet over medium-high heat. Add tallow or fat. Once hot, place the thighs *skin-side down* and cook undisturbed for **7–10 minutes**, until the skin is golden brown and crispy.

4. **Finish in the Oven**

Transfer the skillet to the oven (still skin-side down) and bake for **15–20 minutes** until the internal temperature hits 175°F (80°C).

5. **Rest and Serve**

Remove from the oven, flip thighs skin-side up, and let rest for 5 minutes before serving.

Air Fryer Method (Optional):

- Preheat air fryer to **400°F (200°C)**.
- Pat thighs dry and season.
- Place skin-side down for 12 minutes, then flip and cook another 10–12 minutes until skin is crisp and internal temp is 175°F.

Tips:

- Dry skin = crisp skin. Don't skip the paper towel step.
- Don't move the chicken while searing—it needs time to form that crackly crust.

Perfect with a drizzle of leftover chicken fat or paired with bone broth for a simple, nourishing carnivore meal.

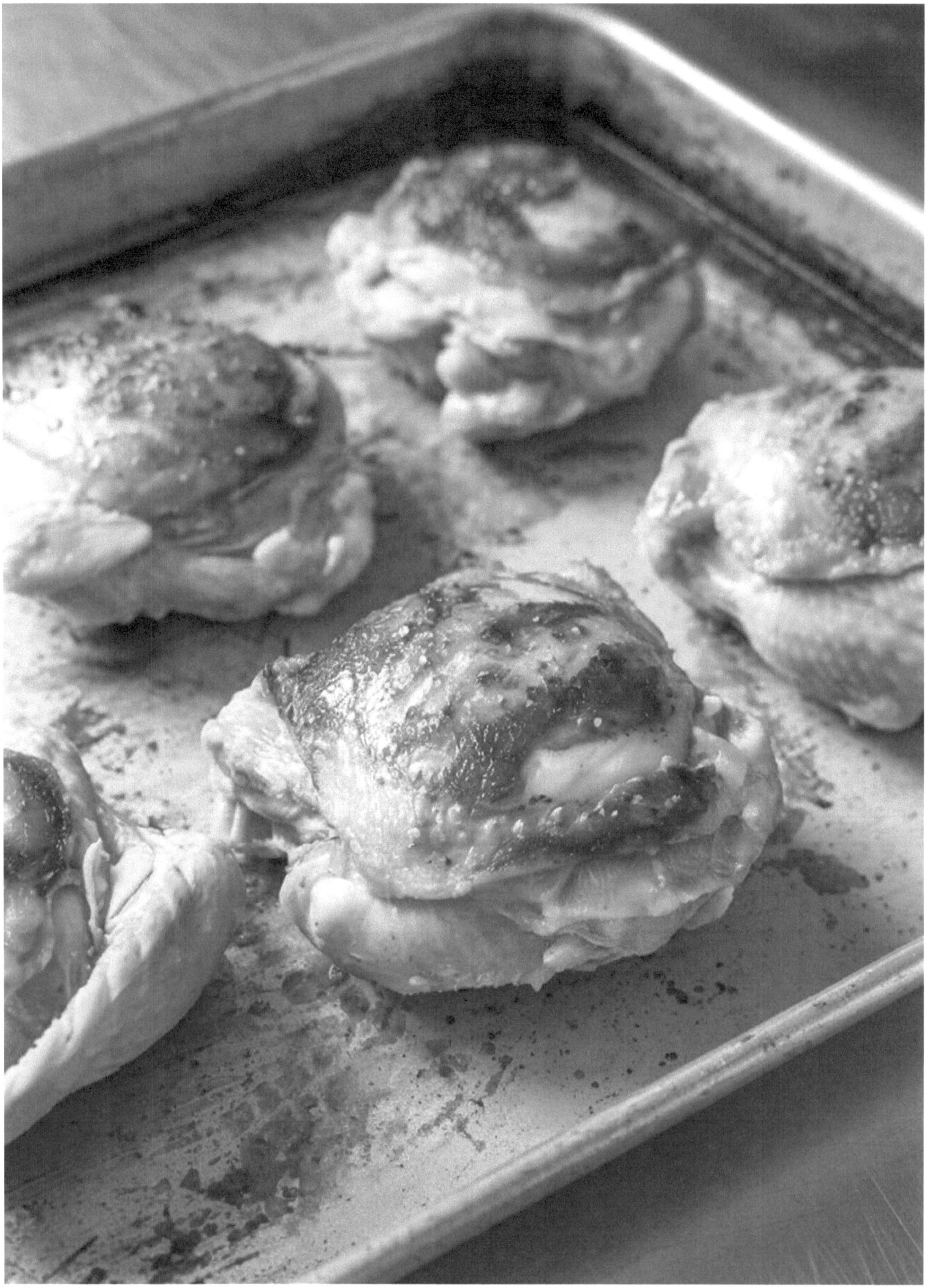

Air Fryer Shrimp

Here's a quick and tasty recipe for **Air Fryer Shrimp**—crispy, juicy, and ready in under 10 minutes. No breadcrumbs, no carbs, just pure protein and flavor.

Air Fryer Shrimp

Yield: 2 servings

Prep Time: 5 minutes

Cook Time: 6–8 minutes

Total Time: ~10–12 minutes

Ingredients:

- 1 lb **raw shrimp**, peeled and deveined (tail on or off)
- 1 tbsp **melted butter**, ghee, or beef tallow
- 1 tsp **sea salt**
- Optional: ½ tsp **garlic powder**, smoked salt, or paprika (omit for strict carnivore)

Instructions:

1. **Preheat Air Fryer**

Set to **400°F (200°C)** and let it preheat for 2–3 minutes.

2. **Prepare the Shrimp**

Pat shrimp dry with paper towels. In a bowl, toss shrimp with melted fat and sea salt until well coated. Add optional seasonings if desired.

3. **Air Fry**

Place shrimp in a single layer in the air fryer basket (don't overcrowd).

Cook for **6–8 minutes**, shaking the basket halfway through. Shrimp are done when pink, curled, and slightly golden at the edges.

4. **Serve Immediately**

Enjoy hot, with a side of bone broth or dipped in melted butter or beef tallow for extra fat.

Tips:

- For extra crispiness, cook for 1 extra minute at the end.
- Great for meal prep—these reheat well and pair nicely with eggs, steak, or liver pâté.

Simple, fast, and protein-packed—this air fryer shrimp is perfect for when you want something light but satisfying on a carnivore plan.

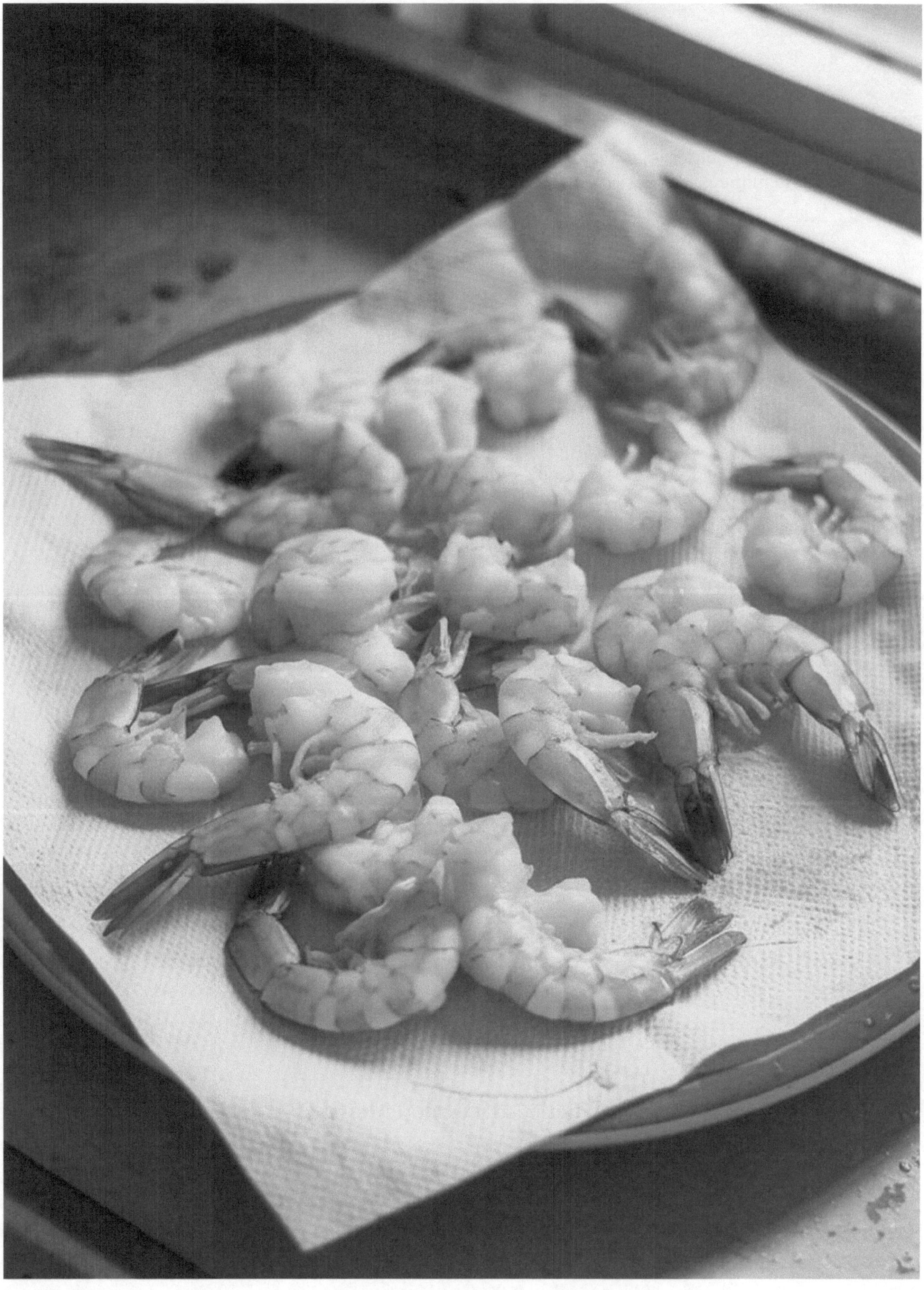

Salmon Bites

Here's a delicious, nutrient-rich recipe for **Salmon Bites**—crispy on the outside, buttery on the inside, and ready in minutes. Perfect as a snack, main dish, or fatty side for leaner meats.

Salmon Bites

Yield: 2–3 servings

Prep Time: 5 minutes

Cook Time: 8–10 minutes

Total Time: ~15 minutes

Ingredients:

- 1 lb **skinless salmon fillet**, cut into 1-inch cubes
- 1 tbsp **butter**, ghee, or beef tallow (for searing)
- 1 tsp **sea salt**
- Optional: ½ tsp **lemon juice**, smoked salt, or garlic powder (omit for strict carnivore)

Instructions (Stovetop Method):

1. **Prepare the Salmon**

Pat salmon cubes dry with paper towels for better sear. Season with salt and optional extras if desired.

2. Heat the Pan

In a large skillet, heat butter or tallow over medium-high heat until shimmering.

3. Sear the Bites

Add salmon pieces in a single layer. Sear for **2–3 minutes per side**, turning gently with tongs until all sides are golden and the centers are just cooked through.

4. Serve Hot

Spoon any leftover pan fat over the top for extra flavor. Eat as-is or pair with eggs or bone broth.

Air Fryer Option:

- Preheat air fryer to **400°F (200°C)**.
- Toss salmon bites in melted fat and salt.
- Air fry for **6–8 minutes**, shaking halfway through.

Tips:

- For fattier bites, use wild-caught **king salmon** or **Atlantic salmon**.
- Avoid overcooking—salmon should be tender, not dry.

> High in omega-3s and quick to prep, these salmon bites are a perfect carnivore-friendly change of pace from red meat.

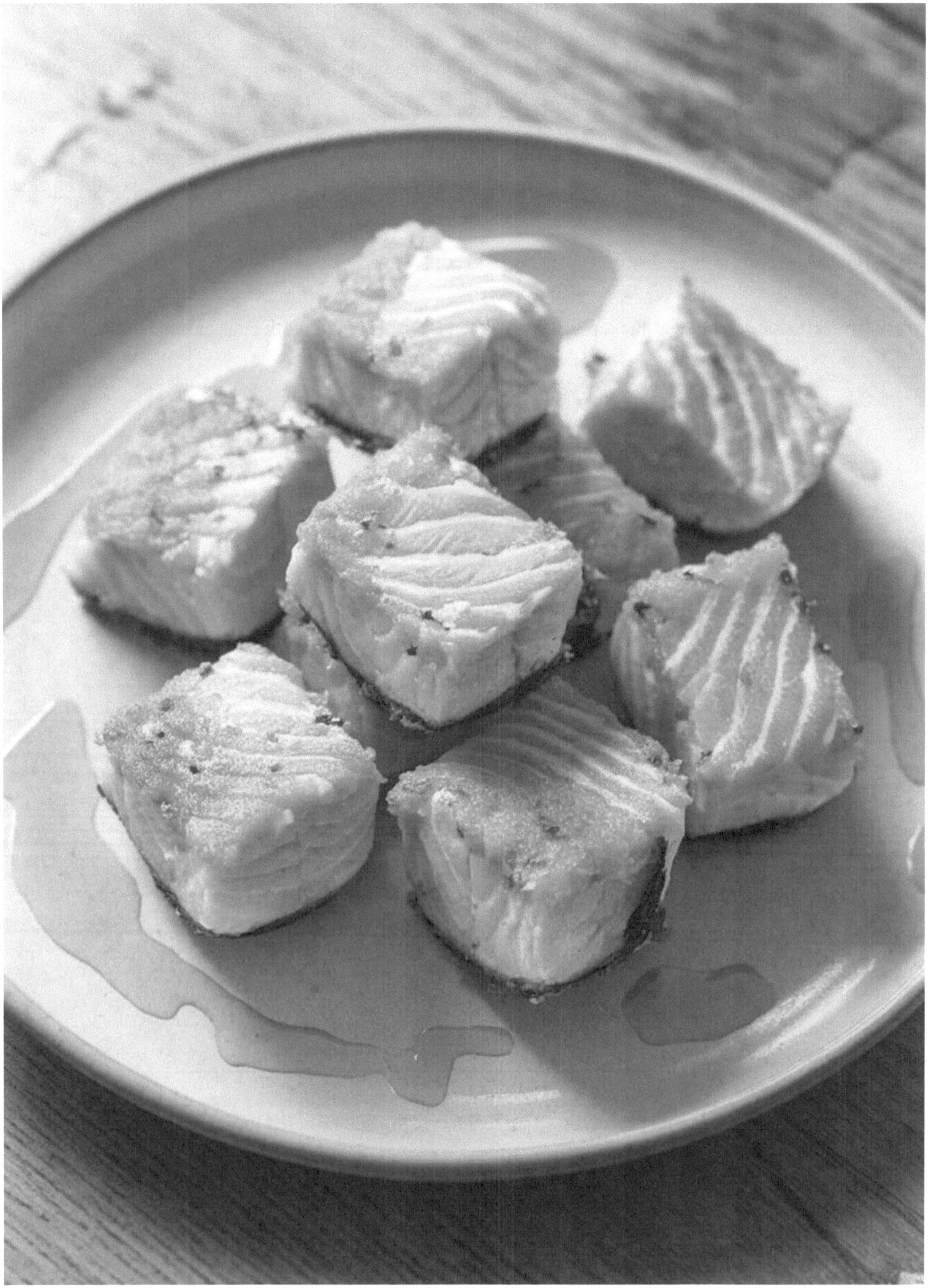

Pan-Seared Chicken Breast

Here's a juicy and flavorful **Pan-Seared Chicken Breast** recipe, done carnivore-style—no flour, no fillers, just pure protein, salt, and fat. Perfect for a quick lunch or dinner when you want something lean but satisfying.

Pan-Seared Chicken Breast (Carnivore Style)

Yield: 2 servings

Prep Time: 5 minutes

Cook Time: 10–12 minutes

Total Time: ~15–20 minutes

Ingredients:

- 2 **boneless, skinless chicken breasts**
- 1½ tsp **sea salt**, divided
- 1 tbsp **beef tallow**, ghee, or butter
- Optional: ½ tsp **garlic powder** or black pepper (omit for strict carnivore)

Instructions:

1. **Prep the Chicken**

Pat the chicken breasts dry with paper towels. Season both sides generously with 1 tsp of salt (and optional garlic powder if using).

2. **Heat the Skillet**

In a cast iron or stainless steel skillet, heat the fat over **medium-high heat** until shimmering.

3. **Sear the First Side**

Place the chicken in the pan and let it cook undisturbed for **5–6 minutes**, or until the bottom develops a deep golden crust. Resist the urge to move it around.

4. **Flip & Finish**

Flip the chicken and reduce heat slightly to medium. Cook another **5–6 minutes**, or until internal temperature reaches **165°F (74°C)**.

5. **Rest Before Serving**

Remove the chicken from the pan, sprinkle with the remaining ½ tsp salt, and let it rest for 5 minutes before slicing. This locks in the juices.

Tips:

- If your chicken is very thick, pound it to an even thickness for faster, even cooking.
- Spoon some of the leftover pan fat over the sliced breast for added flavor and moisture.

> Simple, clean, and protein-packed—this pan-seared chicken breast is a carnivore staple when you want a quick, lean meal with bold flavor.

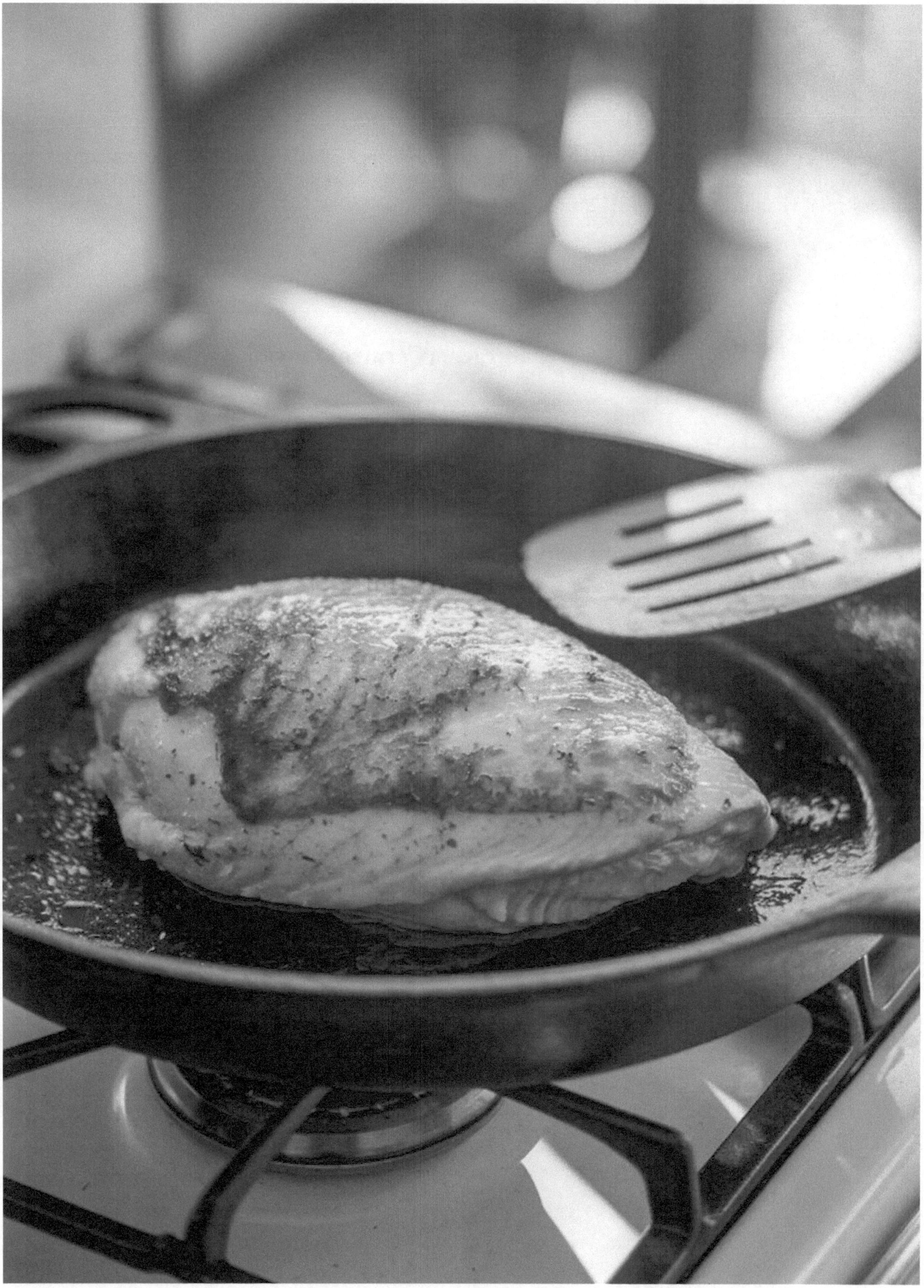

Hidden Liver Burgers

Here's a perfect beginner-friendly **Hidden Liver Burger** recipe—ideal for sneaking nutrient-dense organ meat into your carnivore meals without even tasting it. These burgers are juicy, flavorful, and packed with essential vitamins, especially B12, iron, and vitamin A.

Hidden Liver Burgers (Carnivore Style)

Yield: 4 patties

Prep Time: 10 minutes

Cook Time: 8–10 minutes

Total Time: ~20 minutes

Ingredients:

- 1 lb **ground beef** (80/20 preferred)
- 2–3 oz **beef liver**, finely minced or blended
- 1 tsp **sea salt**
- 1 tbsp **beef tallow** or butter (for cooking)
- Optional: ½ tsp garlic powder or smoked salt (omit for strict carnivore)

Instructions:

1. **Prep the Liver**

If using whole liver, trim membranes and blend it in a food processor until smooth. If pre-ground, skip this step. You can freeze liver slightly to make it easier to grate or mince.

2. **Mix the Meat**

In a bowl, combine ground beef, liver, and salt. Mix thoroughly until the liver is fully incorporated but don't overwork it.

3. **Form Patties**

Divide mixture into 4 equal portions and form into burger patties.

4. **Cook the Burgers**

Heat tallow or butter in a skillet over medium-high heat. Cook patties for **3–4 minutes per side**, or until browned and cooked to your desired doneness.

5. **Serve Hot**

Serve plain, or with a fried egg or melted butter on top for added fat.

Tips:

- Start with 10–15% liver by weight to keep the flavor mild.
- Make a large batch and freeze pre-formed patties for quick meals.
- You can use chicken liver for a milder taste if preferred.

These burgers are a delicious way to get the benefits of organ meats without the strong taste—perfect for families, beginners, or anyone easing into nose-to-tail eating.

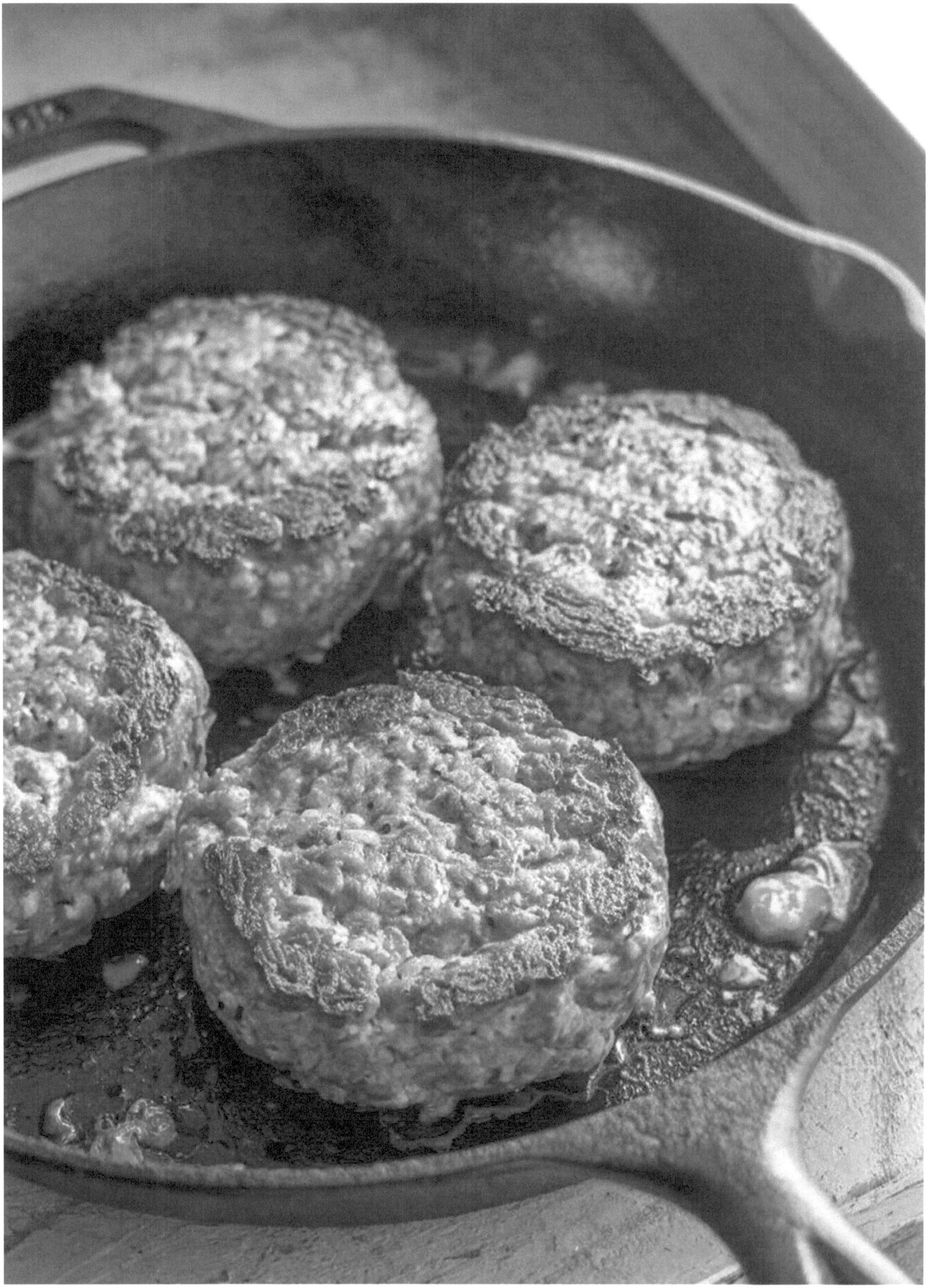

Bacon-Wrapped Chicken Thighs

Here's a savory and satisfying recipe for **Bacon-Wrapped Chicken Thighs (Carnivore Style)**—crispy on the outside, juicy on the inside, and packed with flavor and fat. Perfect for a main course that feels indulgent but stays true to your carnivore goals.

Bacon-Wrapped Chicken Thighs
Yield: 4 servings
Prep Time: 10 minutes
Cook Time: 30–35 minutes
Total Time: ~45 minutes

Ingredients:

- 4 **boneless, skinless chicken thighs**
- 8 slices **bacon** (preferably thin-cut for crispiness)
- 1 tsp **sea salt**
- Optional: ½ tsp **garlic powder** or **black pepper** (omit for strict carnivore)

Instructions:

1. Preheat the Oven

Preheat your oven to **400°F (200°C)**. Line a baking sheet with foil or parchment for easy cleanup. Place a wire rack on top if you have one.

2. Season the Thighs

Pat the chicken thighs dry with paper towels. Season both sides with salt (and optional garlic powder if using).

3. Wrap with Bacon

Wrap each chicken thigh with 2 slices of bacon, slightly overlapping. Tuck the ends underneath or secure with toothpicks if needed.

4. Bake

Place the bacon-wrapped thighs seam-side down on the wire rack or baking sheet. Bake for **30–35 minutes**, or until the internal temperature reaches **175°F (80°C)** and bacon is crisp.

5. Optional Broil

For extra-crispy bacon, broil on high for an additional 2–3 minutes at the end. Watch closely to avoid burning.

6. Rest and Serve

Let the thighs rest for 5 minutes before serving to allow juices to settle.

Tips:

- For fattier flavor, drizzle with melted butter or tallow before serving.
- Can also be cooked in an air fryer at 375°F for 18–20 minutes, flipping halfway.

These bacon-wrapped chicken thighs are rich, hearty, and packed with carnivore-approved flavor—perfect for batch cooking or impressing guests.

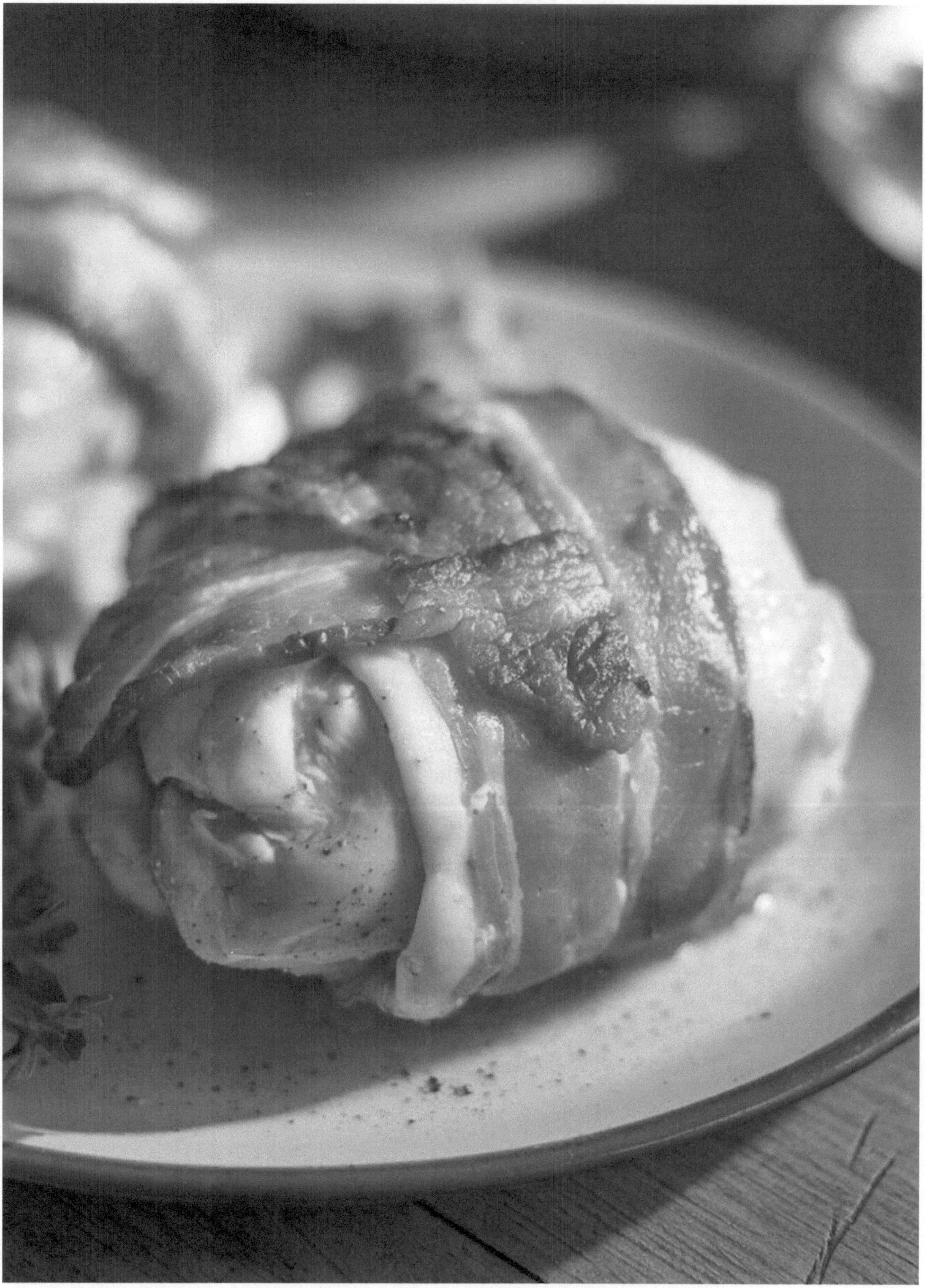

Carnitas

Here's a juicy, fall-apart-tender recipe for **Carnivore Carnitas**—a pork-lover's dream with crispy edges and rich, meaty flavor, all made without citrus, sugar, or spices. Just pork, salt, and fat—pure carnivore style.

Carnivore Carnitas

Yield: 6 servings

Prep Time: 10 minutes

Cook Time: 3–4 hours (stovetop or oven) or 90 min (Instant Pot)

Total Time: Varies by method

Ingredients:

- 3–4 lb **pork shoulder** (also called pork butt), cut into large chunks
- 1 tbsp **sea salt**
- 2 tbsp **lard** or **tallow**
- Optional: 1 tsp **garlic powder** (omit for strict carnivore)
- 1 cup **bone broth** or water (for stovetop or pressure cooker)

Instructions (Stovetop or Oven Method):

1. **Brown the Pork**

Heat lard or tallow in a large Dutch oven over medium-high heat. Add pork chunks and sear until browned on all sides. Do it in batches if needed.

2. **Add Broth & Simmer**

Add bone broth and salt. Cover and reduce heat to low, or transfer to a 300°F (150°C) oven. Cook **3–4 hours**, until pork is fork-tender and falling apart.

3. **Shred the Pork**

Remove lid, increase heat to medium-high, and continue cooking uncovered to evaporate liquid. Stir occasionally to crisp up the shredded meat in its own rendered fat.

4. **Serve Crispy**

For even more crispiness, transfer to a baking sheet and broil for 5 minutes, then stir and broil another 3–5 minutes.

Instant Pot Method:

- Follow steps 1 and 2 above in sauté mode.
- Pressure cook on high for **90 minutes**, natural release 10 minutes.
- Shred, then crisp up in a skillet or under the broiler.

Tips:

- Serve with extra melted lard or tallow for richness.
- Store leftovers in the fat to keep them moist and flavorful.

> These carnitas are 100% carnivore-approved—crispy, juicy, and packed with slow-cooked porky goodness.

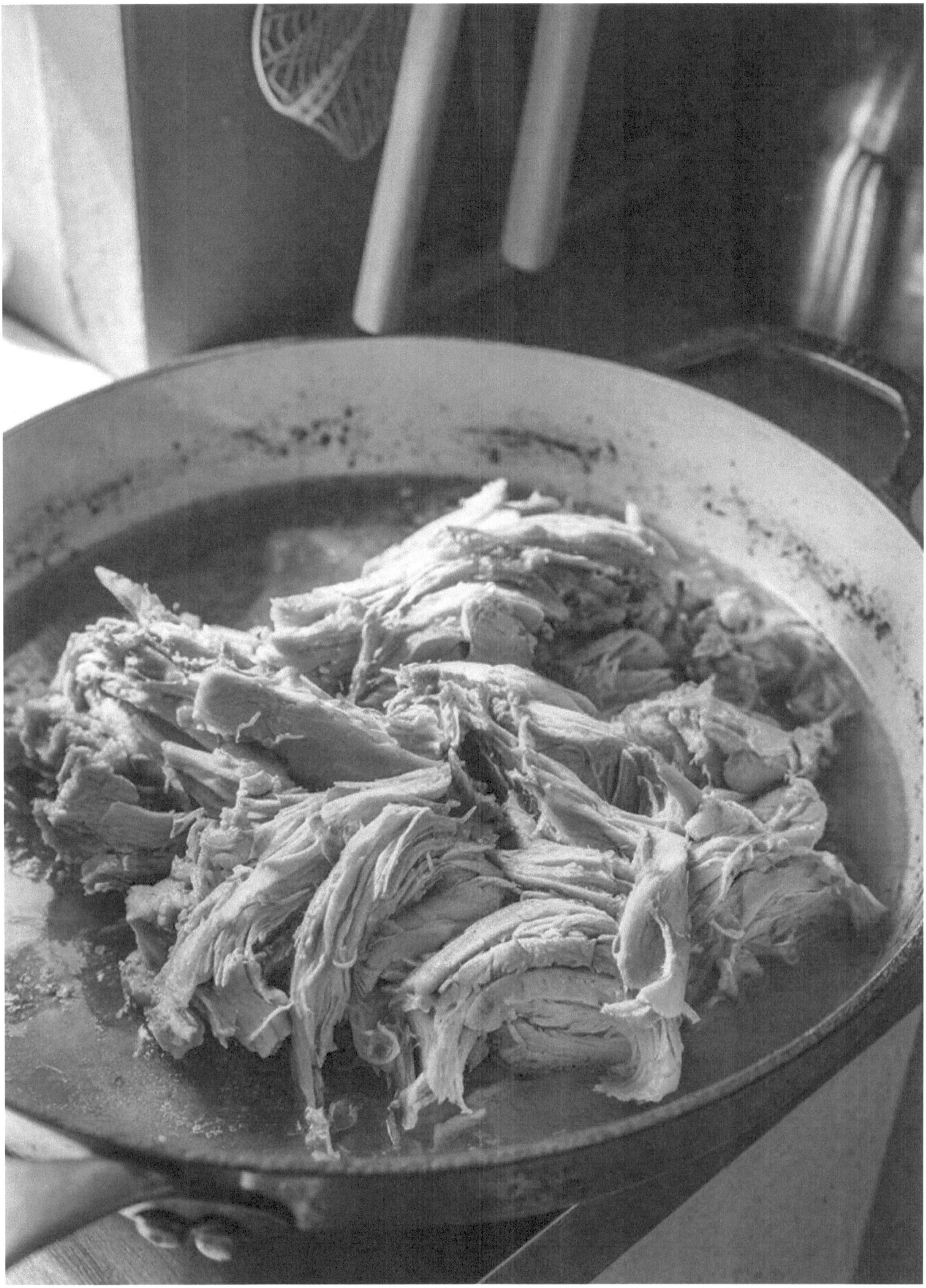

Kofta Meatballs

Here's a simple and flavorful recipe for **Kofta Meatballs (Carnivore Style)**—inspired by Middle Eastern kofta but stripped down to the essentials for a zero-carb, all-meat meal. These meatballs are juicy, rich, and perfect for batch cooking or meal prep.

Carnivore Kofta Meatballs
Yield: 12–14 meatballs (3–4 servings)
Prep Time: 10 minutes
Cook Time: 15–20 minutes
Total Time: ~30 minutes

Ingredients:

- 1 lb **ground lamb** (or beef or a 50/50 mix)
- 2 oz **beef liver**, finely minced or blended *(optional for extra nutrients)*
- 1 tsp **sea salt**
- 1 tbsp **beef tallow**, butter, or ghee (for cooking)
- Optional: ½ tsp **cumin**, **garlic powder**, or **cinnamon** (omit for strict carnivore)

Instructions:

1. **Mix the Meat**

In a bowl, combine ground lamb (or beef), minced liver if using, and salt. Add optional spices for a traditional kofta flavor if desired.

2. **Form the Meatballs**

Roll mixture into 1½-inch balls. You should get 12–14 meatballs.

3. **Cook in Skillet**

Heat fat in a large skillet over medium heat. Add meatballs in a single layer and cook for **8–10 minutes**, turning occasionally, until browned on all sides and cooked through.

4. **Optional Finish**

For extra crispness, place cooked meatballs on a baking sheet and broil for 2–3 minutes.

5. **Serve Hot**

Drizzle with pan juices or extra melted tallow. Pairs well with eggs, broth, or a side of bone marrow.

Tips:

- Ground lamb gives a rich, authentic kofta taste, but beef works great too.
- Liver adds depth and nutrition but can be left out for a milder flavor.
- Make a double batch and freeze extras for easy meals.

These carnivore kofta meatballs are protein-packed,
rich in fat, and bursting with meaty flavor—even without herbs or carbs.

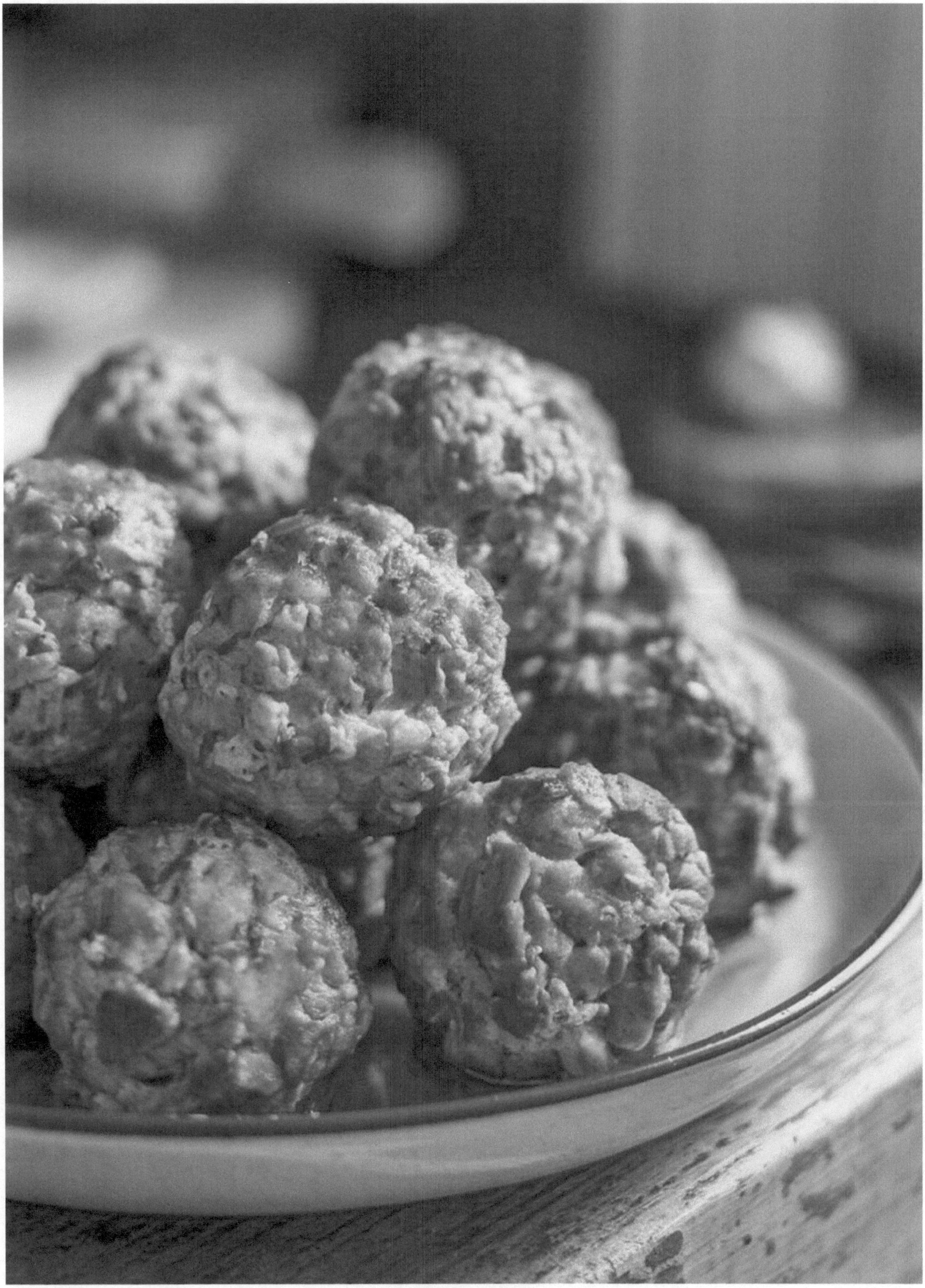

Baked Bacon

Here's a no-mess, foolproof method for **Baked Bacon (Carnivore Style)**—perfectly crispy strips every time without the stovetop splatter. Great for meal prep, snack trays, or adding fat to lean cuts.

Baked Bacon

Yield: 4 servings

Prep Time: 5 minutes

Cook Time: 18–22 minutes

Total Time: ~25 minutes

Ingredients:

- 1 lb **bacon** (thin or thick-cut, uncured preferred)
- Optional: **parchment paper** or **foil** for easier cleanup

Instructions:

1. **Preheat Oven**

Set oven to **400°F (200°C)**. Line a baking sheet with foil or parchment. Place a wire rack on top if you prefer extra-crispy bacon, or lay bacon directly on the sheet for fattier, chewier strips.

2. **Arrange the Bacon**

Lay the bacon slices flat in a single layer without overlapping. You may need two trays depending on size.

3. **Bake**

Bake for **18–22 minutes**, depending on thickness and desired crispiness:

- Thin-cut: 16–18 minutes
- Thick-cut: 20–24 minutes

Check around the 15-minute mark and rotate trays if using two.

4. **Cool & Drain**

Remove from oven and transfer bacon to a paper towel-lined plate or rack to drain excess fat (or eat it straight for max fat retention).

5. **Serve or Store**

Serve hot or store in a sealed container in the fridge for up to 5 days. Reheat in an air fryer, skillet, or oven.

Tips:

- Save the rendered bacon fat to cook eggs, ground beef, or pan-sear steak.
- Want it extra crunchy? Broil for the last 1–2 minutes—watch closely!

Simple, crispy, and carnivore-perfect—baked bacon is a meal prep staple that delivers every time.

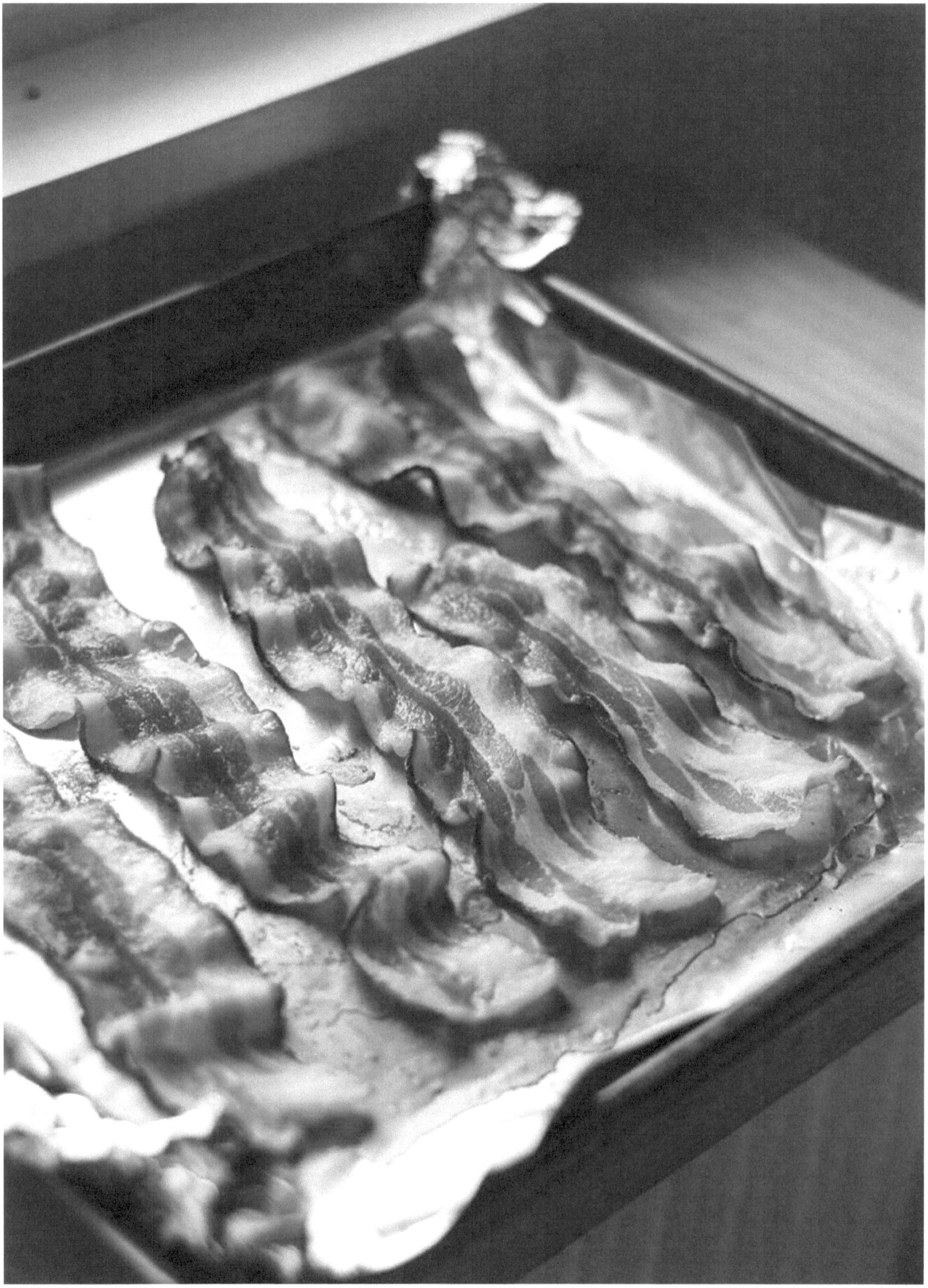

Creamy Chicken Casserole

Here's a **Carnivore-Adapted Creamy Chicken Casserole** recipe—with a rich, dairy-based filling and a crunchy topping. Since panko breadcrumbs aren't carnivore-friendly, we'll swap in a crispy pork rind or cheese crust that gives the same crunch and satisfaction—without any carbs.

Creamy Chicken Casserole (Carnivore Style)

Yield: 4–6 servings

Prep Time: 15 minutes

Cook Time: 25–30 minutes

Total Time: ~45 minutes

Ingredients:

For the Creamy Base:

- 2–3 cups **shredded cooked chicken** (thighs or breast)
- ¾ cup **heavy cream**
- ½ cup **cream cheese**, softened
- ½ cup **shredded hard cheese** (cheddar, gouda, or parmesan)
- 1 tsp **sea salt**
- Optional: ½ tsp **garlic powder**, ¼ tsp **white pepper** (omit for strict carnivore)

For the Crunchy Topping:

- 1 cup **crushed pork rinds**
- OR ½ cup **shredded parmesan** (or a mix of both)
- 2 tbsp **butter** or **tallow**, melted

Instructions:

1. Preheat Oven

Preheat to **375°F (190°C)** and grease a small casserole dish with butter or tallow.

2. Make the Creamy Base

In a saucepan over medium heat, combine heavy cream and cream cheese. Stir until melted and smooth. Add shredded cheese and salt, stirring until the sauce is thick and creamy.

3. Assemble the Casserole

In a bowl, toss the shredded chicken with the cheese sauce until fully coated. Spread evenly into the prepared dish.

4. Add Crunchy Topping

Mix crushed pork rinds or parmesan with melted butter or tallow. Sprinkle evenly over the top of the casserole.

5. Bake

Bake uncovered for **25–30 minutes**, until the top is golden and bubbling.

6. Cool & Serve

Let rest for 5–10 minutes before serving to allow the sauce to thicken.

Tips:

- Use rotisserie chicken (skin removed) for extra flavor and ease.
- Add a few dollops of bone marrow before baking for a nutritional boost.
- Leftovers reheat beautifully in the oven or air fryer.

> This creamy chicken casserole gives you all the comfort of classic home cooking—without the carbs or plant-based ingredients.

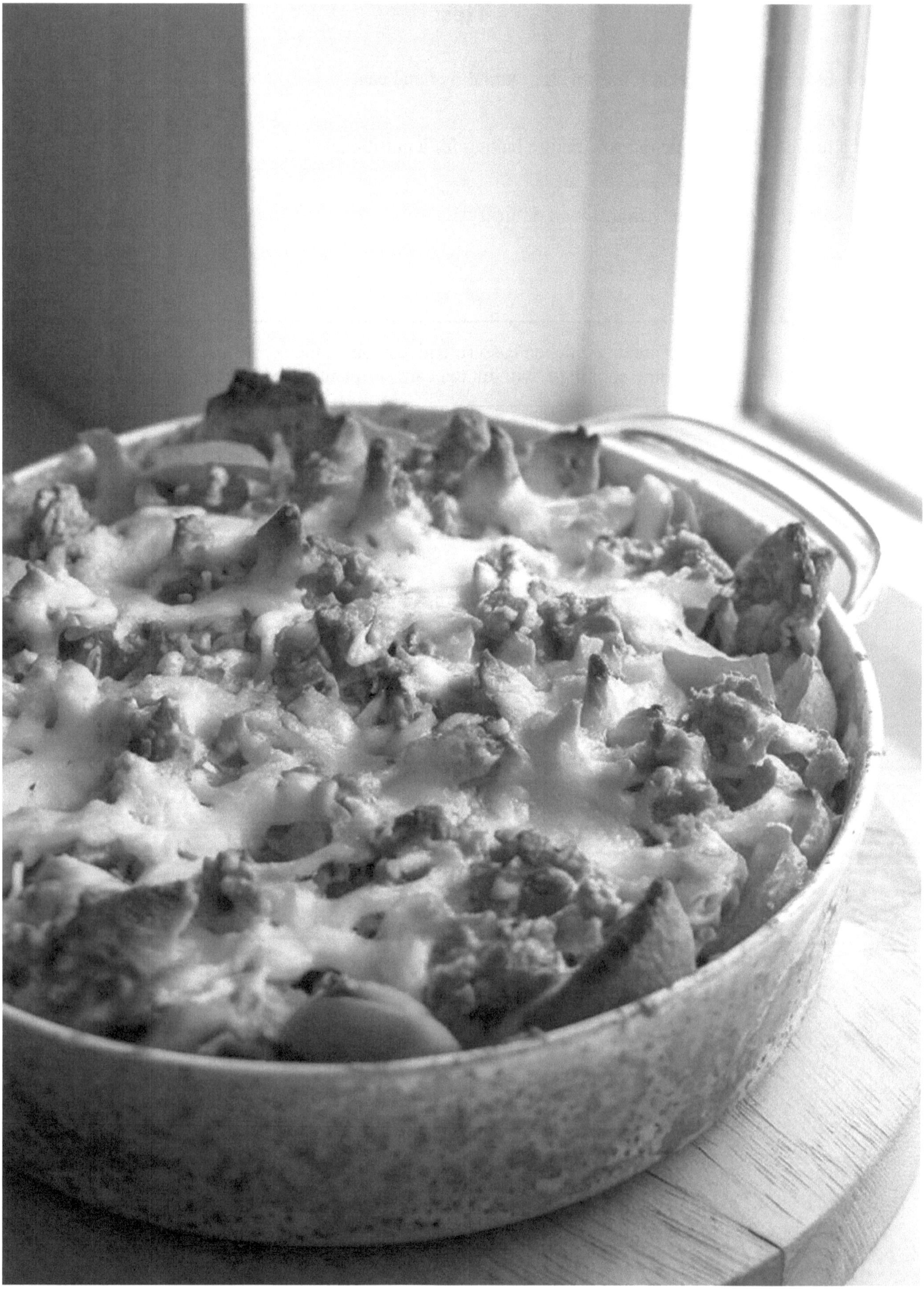

Meatloaf

Here's a slightly altered, richer version of your **Carnivore Meatloaf** recipe—boosted for flavor, fat content, and tenderness, while staying true to carnivore principles. We'll keep the texture moist and satisfying while leaning into deeper umami from a touch of organ meat (optional) and fat.

Ultimate Carnivore Meatloaf

Yield: 6–8 servings

Prep Time: 10 minutes

Cook Time: 50–60 minutes

Total Time: ~1 hour 10 minutes

Ingredients:

- 2 lbs **ground beef** (80/20 or fattier)
- 2 **large eggs**
- ¼ cup **heavy cream**
- ½ cup **pork panko** (crushed pork rinds)
- 1 tbsp **beef liver**, finely grated or puréed *(optional but highly nutritious)*
- 1 tsp **sea salt**
- ½ tsp **onion powder** or **garlic powder** *(optional for non-strict carnivore)*

- 1 tbsp **beef tallow** or **butter**, melted (plus extra for greasing)

Instructions:

1. **Preheat Oven**

Preheat to **350°F (175°C)**. Grease a loaf pan or line with parchment paper.

2. **Mix the Ingredients**

In a large bowl, combine all ingredients. Use your hands to gently mix until just combined—don't overwork the meat.

3. **Shape the Loaf**

Transfer mixture into the prepared loaf pan and smooth the top. Optional: score the top with a knife for more crust.

4. **Bake**

Bake uncovered for **50–60 minutes**, or until internal temp reaches **160°F (71°C)**. For a firmer crust, broil the top for 3–5 minutes at the end.

5. **Rest & Serve**

Let rest 10 minutes before slicing. Serve with melted butter, extra tallow drizzled on top, or even a fried egg.

Tips:

- Add ¼ cup shredded cheddar for a cheesier version.
- Ground pork can be substituted for half the beef to change up the flavor and fat ratio.

> This variation delivers rich flavor, juicy texture,
> and sneaky nutrition—with just the right balance of meat and fat.

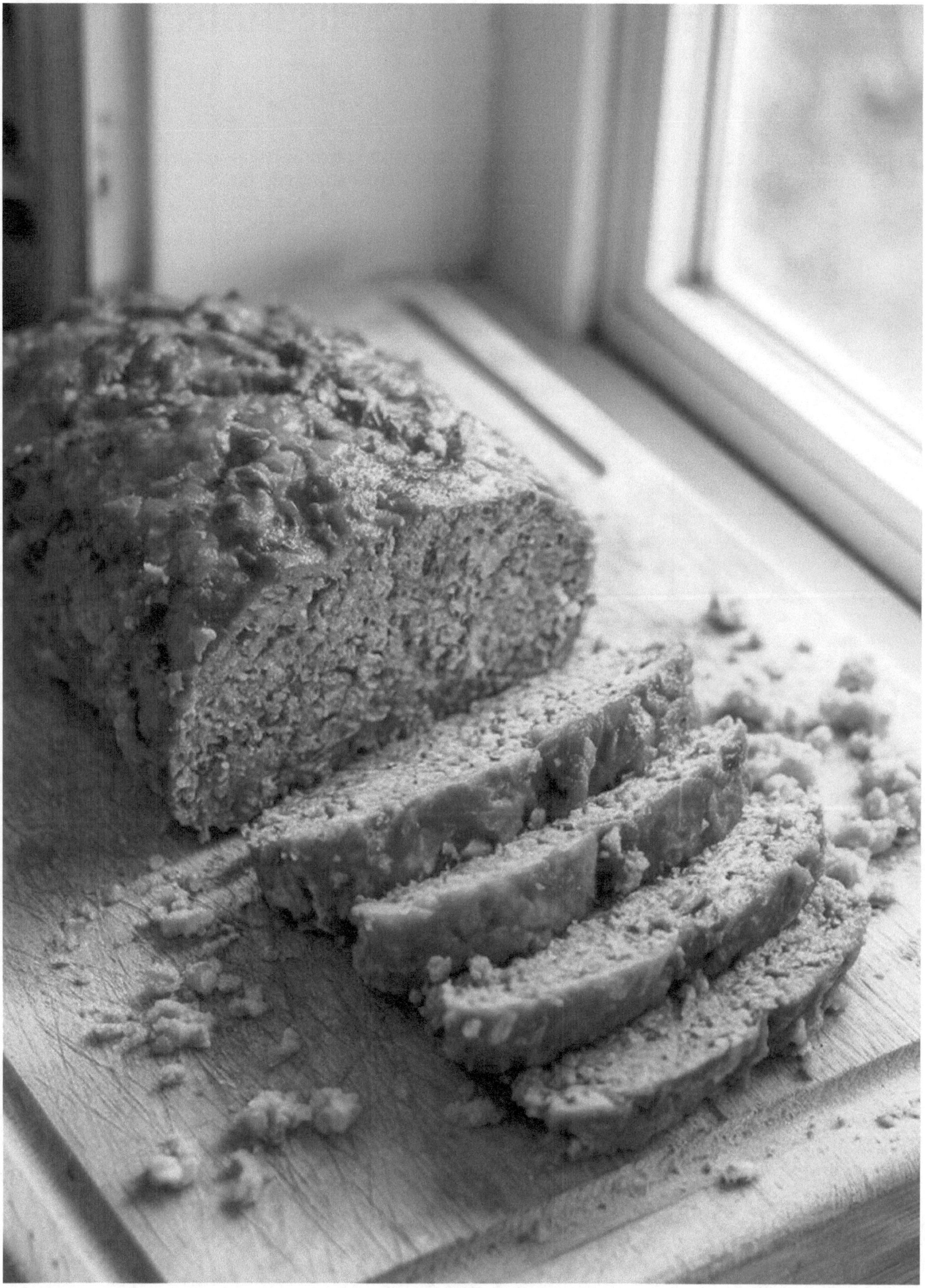

Lamb Chops with Garlic Butter

Here's a quick and flavorful recipe for Lamb Chops with Garlic Butter—tender, juicy, and ready in minutes. Perfectly seared and basted in rich, carnivore-approved fat.

Lamb Chops with Garlic Butter
Yield: 2 servings
Prep Time: 5 minutes
Cook Time: 8–10 minutes
Total Time: ~15 minutes

Ingredients:

- 4 lamb chops (about 1 inch thick)
- 2 tbsp butter, ghee, or beef tallow
- 2 cloves garlic, minced (optional for less strict carnivore)
- 1 tsp sea salt
- ½ tsp black pepper (omit for strict carnivore)

Instructions:

1. **Prepare the Lamb**

Pat lamb chops dry with paper towels. Season generously with sea salt (and pepper if using).

2. **Heat the Pan**

In a cast iron skillet, melt butter or tallow over medium-high heat until sizzling.

3. **Sear the Chops**

Add lamb chops and sear 3–4 minutes per side until golden brown and crusted.

4. **Add Garlic Butter**

Reduce heat to medium. Add minced garlic (if using) and baste chops with melted butter for 1–2 minutes until fragrant.

5. **Rest and Serve**

Remove from heat, let rest for 5 minutes, then serve with a drizzle of pan juices.

Tips:

- For extra richness, add a dollop of whipped bone marrow butter on top before serving.
- Works just as well with lamb loin chops or rib chops.
- Pair with crispy bacon or a simple egg scramble for a full carnivore plate.

Juicy, buttery, and packed with flavor—these lamb chops are a perfect high-fat, high-protein carnivore meal.

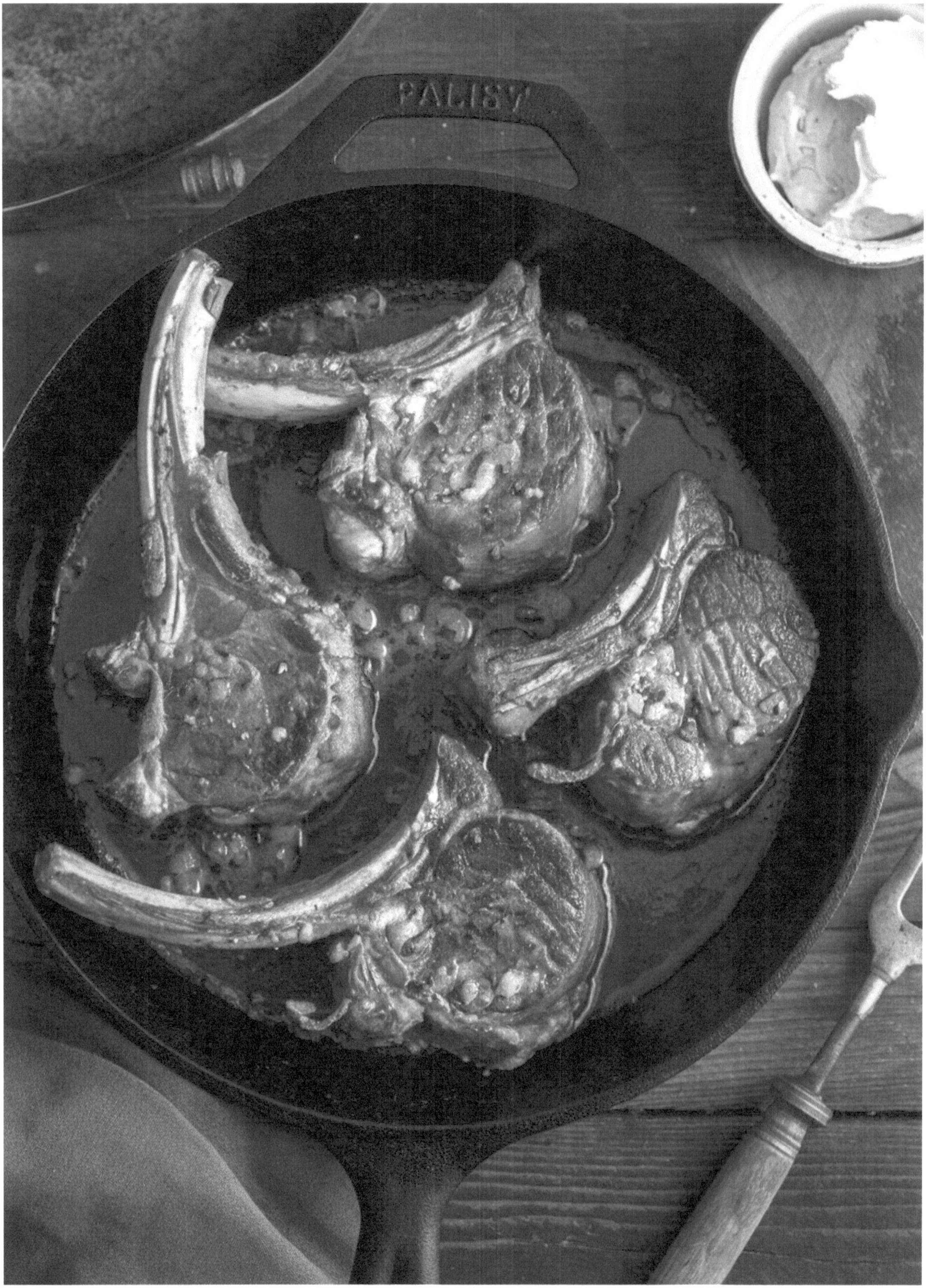
PALISV

Carnivore Chili (No Beans, No Tomatoes)

Yield: 4–6 servings

Prep Time: 10 minutes

Cook Time: 45–60 minutes

Total Time: ~1 hour 10 minutes

Ingredients:

- 2 lbs **ground beef** (80/20 or fattier)
- ½ lb **ground pork** or **ground lamb** (optional for variety)
- 2 tbsp **beef tallow** or **butter**
- 2 tsp **sea salt**
- 1 tsp **smoked salt** or **bacon fat** (optional, for smoky flavor)
- 1 tsp **garlic powder** (optional)
- 1 cup **beef bone broth**

Optional Add-ins (non-strict carnivore):

- ½ tsp **paprika**, **cumin**, or **onion powder**
- 2 tbsp **cream cheese** or **cheddar**, stirred in at the end for creaminess

Instructions:

1. **Brown the Meat**

Heat tallow in a heavy-bottomed pot or Dutch oven over medium heat. Add ground beef (and pork/lamb if using). Cook until browned, breaking up the meat as it cooks.

2. **Season**

Add sea salt and any optional seasonings. Stir to combine. Cook for another 2–3 minutes to allow flavors to develop.

3. **Simmer**

Pour in bone broth and bring to a light simmer. Reduce heat to low, cover partially, and simmer for **30–45 minutes**, stirring occasionally.

4. **Reduce to Thicken**

Uncover and simmer another **10–15 minutes** to thicken. If it reduces too much, add a splash more broth or fat.

5. **Serve Hot**

Spoon into bowls and top with a drizzle of melted butter, shredded cheese (if tolerated), or a fried egg for added fat.

Tips:

- For a chunkier texture, mix in chopped cooked brisket or shredded pot roast.
- To freeze, let cool completely and store in airtight containers.

This carnivore chili is cozy, filling, and
full of meaty goodness—no plants required.

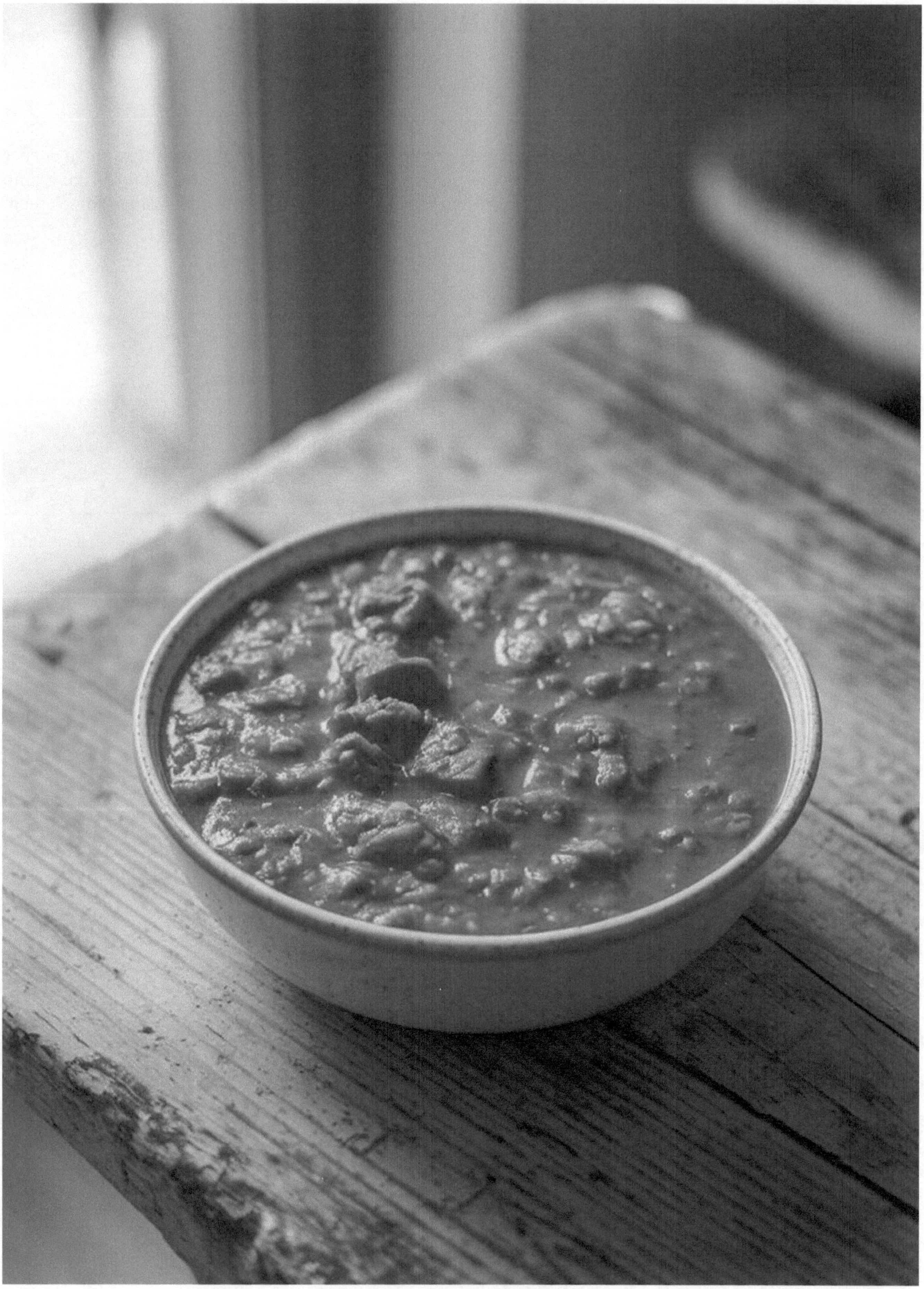

Carnivore Bread

Here's an altered version of your **Carnivore Bread** recipe—slightly adjusted for richer texture, a deeper savory flavor, and more fat to support carnivore macros. It keeps that moist, banana-bread-like crumb but leans even more into buttery, satisfying bites. We'll use a bit less cottage cheese and swap in some cream cheese for extra richness and structure.

Buttery Carnivore Bread (Toasts Like a Dream)

Yield: 1 loaf (about 22 slices, 11 servings)

Prep Time: 10 minutes

Cook Time: 55–60 minutes

Total Time: ~1 hour 10 minutes

Ingredients:

- 12 **large eggs**
- 1 cup **full-fat cottage cheese**
- ½ cup **cream cheese**, softened
- 2 cups (180 g) **pork panko**
- ½ cup (1 stick) **salted butter**, melted
- Optional: ½ tsp **baking powder** (for fluffier lift)

Instructions:

1. **Preheat Oven**

Preheat to **375°F (190°C)**. Line a **9x5-inch loaf pan** with parchment paper, letting it hang over the edges for easy lifting.

2. **Blend the Batter**

In a food processor, blend the eggs, cottage cheese, cream cheese, pork panko, and melted butter until smooth and thick. Scrape down sides as needed. Add baking powder if using and pulse once more.

3. **Bake**

Pour the batter into the prepared pan. Bake for **55–60 minutes**, or until golden brown on top and a toothpick inserted in the center comes out clean.

4. **Cool Completely**

Let cool 10–15 minutes before lifting out. Cool completely before slicing for clean cuts and best texture.

Serving Notes:

- **Toasting (Highly Recommended):**

Toast in an air fryer at **425°F** for **10 minutes**, flipping halfway.

Or pan-fry slices in butter until golden. Adds a French toast–like texture.

- **Storage:**

Keeps well in the fridge for 4–5 days. Freeze leftover slices for later—just reheat in toaster, skillet, or air fryer straight from frozen.

> This version adds richness, a slightly firmer structure, and better toasting performance while staying 100% carnivore-friendly. Great for buttered toast, savory sandwiches, or pan-fried "French toast" style indulgence.

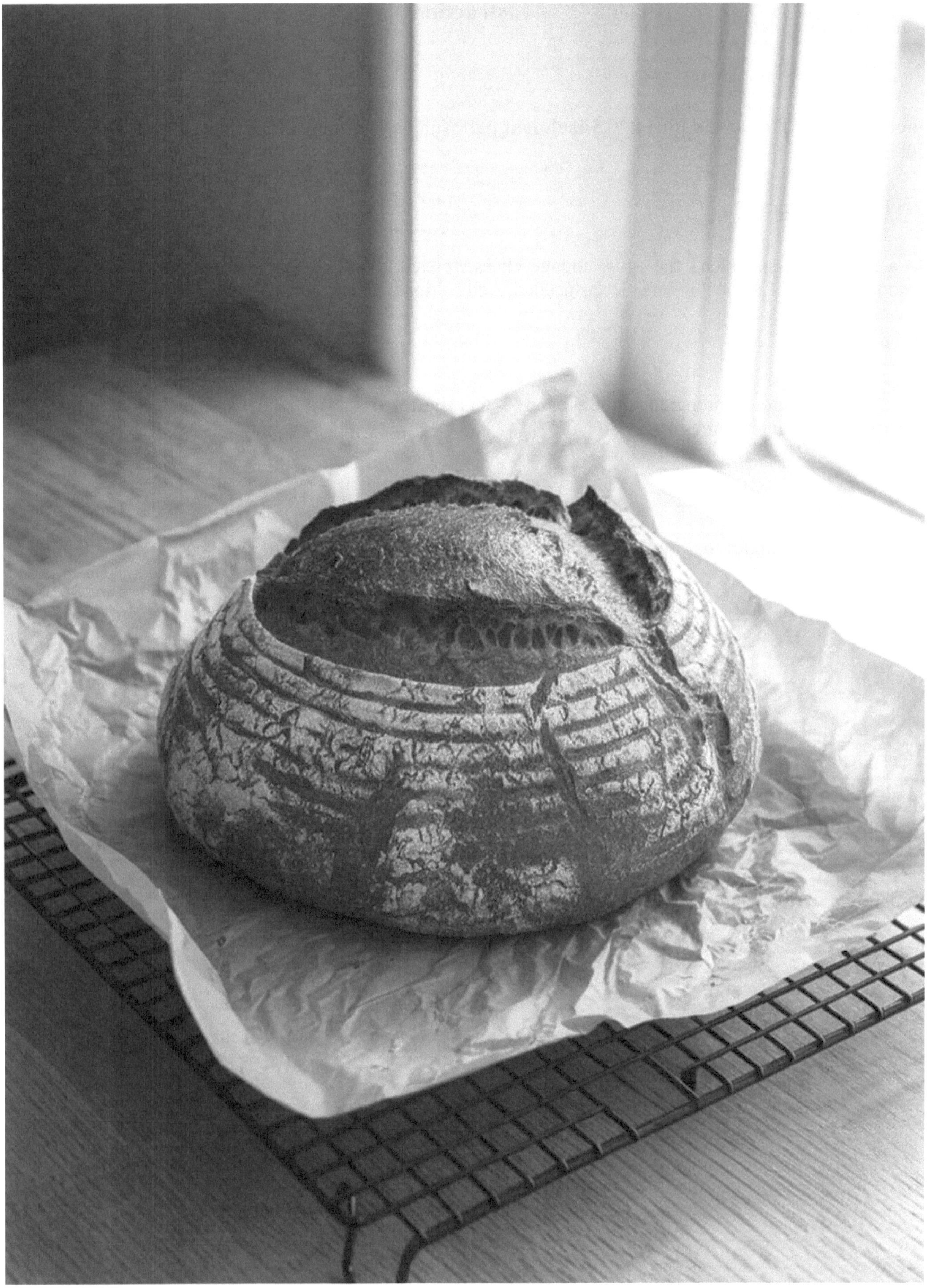

English Muffins

Here's a **Carnivore English Muffins**. The texture is fluffier and less dense, making them ideal for toasting or sandwiching.

Fluffy Carnivore English Muffins

Yield: 6–8 muffins

Prep Time: 5 minutes

Cook Time: 12–15 minutes

Total Time: ~20 minutes

Ingredients:

- 1½ cups (135 g) **pork panko**
- 6 **large eggs**
- 2 tbsp **cream cheese**, softened
- ¼ cup (½ stick) **salted butter**, melted but not hot
- Optional: ½ tsp **baking powder** (for a more bread-like rise)

Instructions:

1. Preheat Oven

Preheat to **375°F (190°C)**. Grease muffin rings or silicone muffin molds and place them on a parchment-lined baking sheet.

2. Blend the Batter

In a blender or food processor, combine eggs, cream cheese, and melted butter. Blend until smooth. Add pork panko (and baking powder, if using), and pulse until fully combined and slightly thickened.

3. Fill the Molds

Pour the batter evenly into muffin molds, filling about ¾ full.

4. Bake

Bake for **12–15 minutes**, or until puffed and golden. A toothpick should come out clean when inserted into the center.

5. Cool & Toast

Let cool slightly before removing. Slice in half and toast in a skillet with butter or in an air fryer for 3–5 minutes at 400°F for a crisp, classic English muffin texture.

Tips:

- For crisper edges, broil the halved muffins for 1–2 minutes after toasting.
- Add a sprinkle of shredded cheese to the tops before baking for a cheesy crust (optional for less strict carnivore).

> These muffins are light, satisfying, and great as a vehicle for eggs, burgers, or just a swipe of butter.

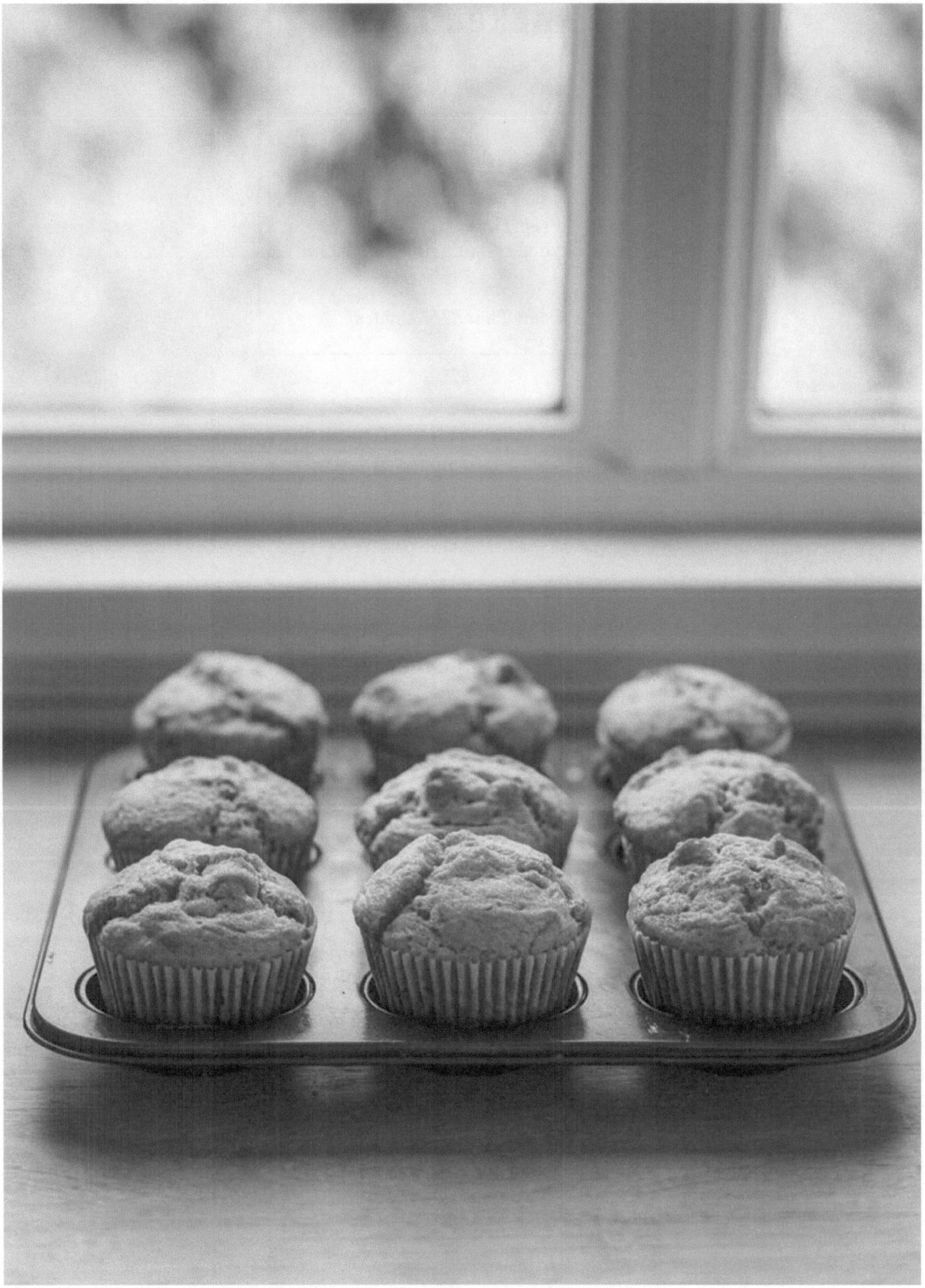

Chicken Flour

Yield: 1 cup

Prep Time: 10 minutes
(not including cooking time for chicken)

Cook Time: 75 minutes

Chicken flour is a surprisingly handy staple—perfect for recipes where you want a fine, high-protein binder or breading alternative without using pork. It's especially useful in dough-style recipes or when you need a light, neutral-flavored base with a dense consistency. Use it as a thickener, coating, or binding ingredient, but be mindful: a little goes a long way.

Ingredients:

- 1½ pounds **boneless, skinless chicken breasts**, cooked and cooled

Special Equipment:

- Food processor or high-powered blender
- Sheet pan
- Parchment paper

Instructions:

1. Preheat Oven

Set oven to **300°F (150°C)**. Line a baking sheet with parchment.

2. Shred the Chicken

Cut cooked chicken into chunks and place into a food processor. Pulse until the texture is finely chopped—almost fluffy, but not paste-like.

3. Dry in Oven

Spread the chopped chicken evenly on the lined sheet pan. Bake for **60 to 75 minutes**, stirring every 20 minutes, until fully dried and lightly browned.

4. Cool & Blend

Once dry and cool, transfer half the dried chicken to a high-powered blender and blitz into a fine powder. Repeat with the remaining half.

Cooking Note:

The best prep method is baking the chicken until it's thoroughly cooked and dry. Bake in an oven at **400°F for 45–50 minutes** or use an air fryer at **400°F for 30 minutes**, depending on thickness. Avoid adding oils or seasonings. Allow the meat to cool fully before processing.

Store in an airtight container in a cool, dry place or in the freezer for long-term use. Use as needed in carnivore doughs, batters, or coating blends.

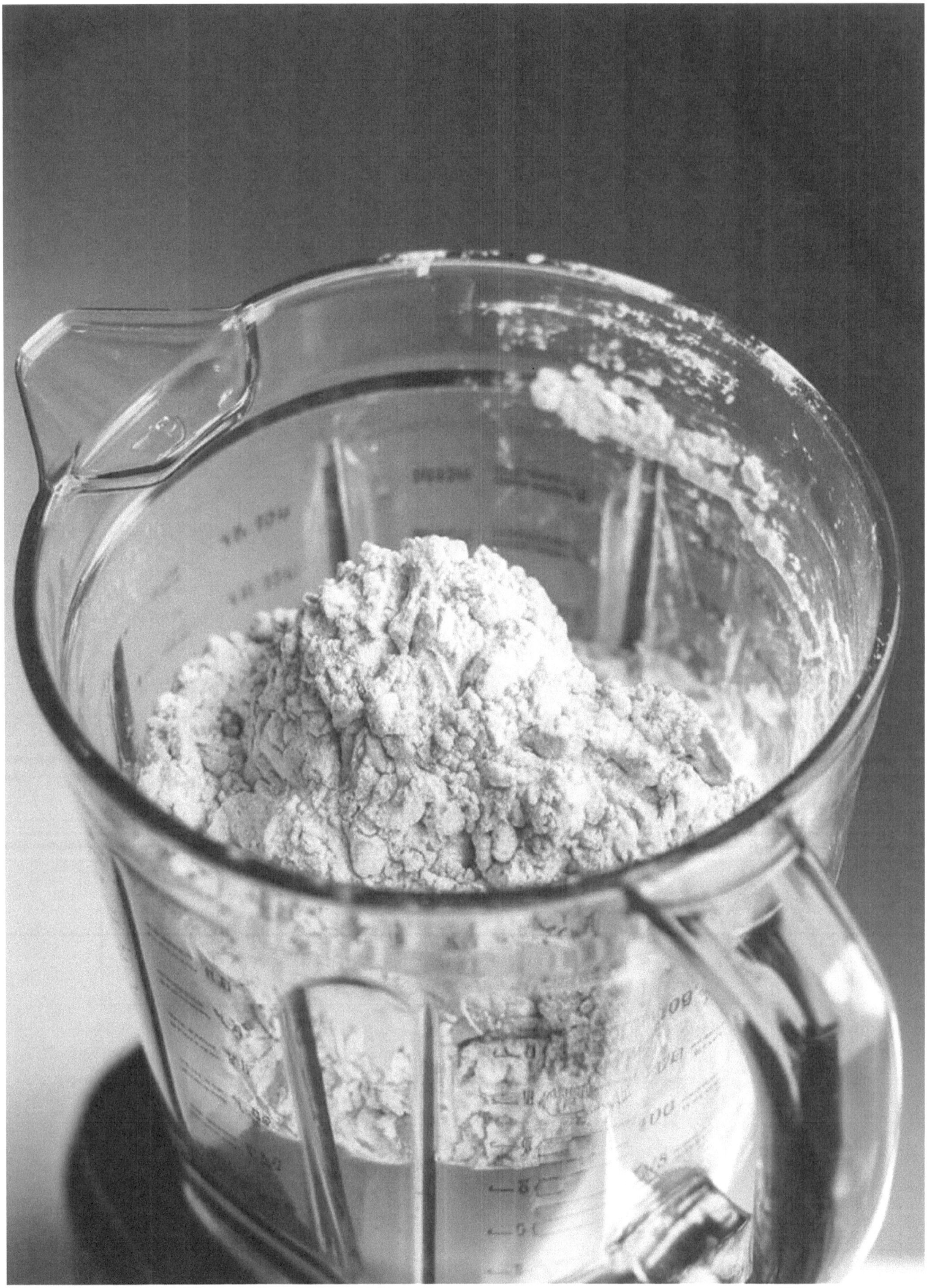

Chicken Noodle Soup (Carnivore Style)

Yield: 2 servings

Prep Time: 5 minutes (not including time to cook chicken or noodles)

Cook Time: 10 minutes

This rich and satisfying soup combines shredded chicken, silky eggs, and tender noodles in a warm, flavorful broth. It's simple, fast, and deeply comforting—perfect for chilly nights or an easy lunch. The eggs give it a naturally creamy texture, and the noodles soak up all the savory goodness. It also stores and reheats well, so don't hesitate to double the batch.

Ingredients:

- 4 cups **chicken broth** (homemade or high-quality store-bought)
- 3 large **eggs**, whisked
- 8 oz **cooked, chopped chicken** (preferably a mix of dark and white meat)
- 1 batch **Egg White Noodles**
- **Kosher salt**, to taste

Instructions:

1. In a medium Dutch oven or soup pot, bring the chicken broth to a low boil over medium-high heat.

2. Lower the heat to medium-low. While gently stirring the broth in a circular motion, slowly drizzle in the whisked eggs to create thin, ribbon-like strands.

3. Stir in the cooked chicken and prepared noodles. Let everything simmer together for 1–2 minutes until heated through.

4. Remove from heat, season with salt to taste, and serve hot.

> **Tip:** This soup keeps well in the fridge for up to 4 days and tastes even better the next day. For best texture, store the noodles separately and add them just before reheating.

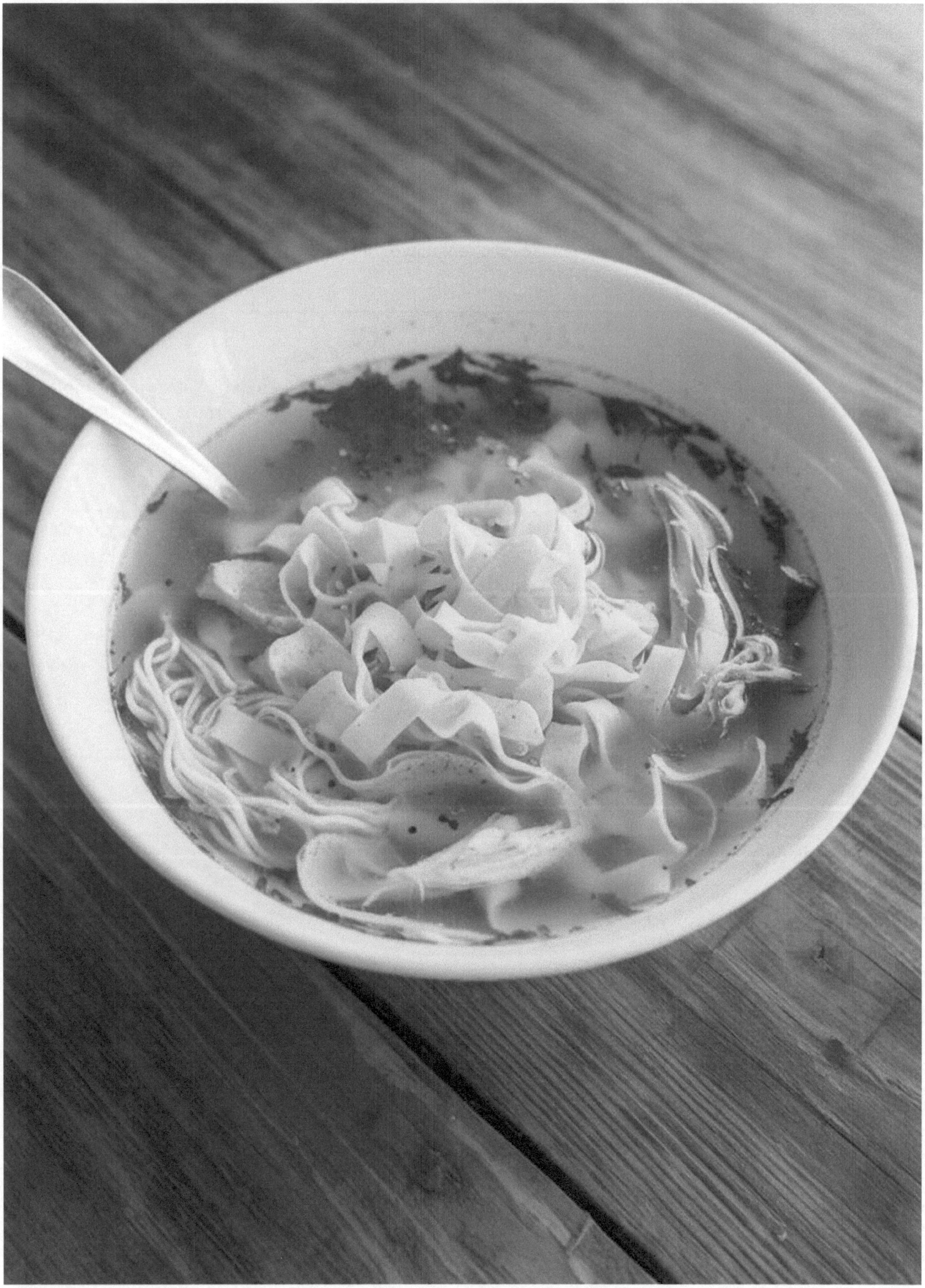

Chicken Salad

Yield: 2 servings

Prep Time: 10 minutes (not including time to make chicken, mayo, or bacon)

This creamy, savory chicken salad is a lunch favorite and meal prep hero. It's satisfying, simple, and perfect for scooping with pork rinds, meat chips, or even eating straight from the bowl. It also stores beautifully in the fridge for several days, making it a reliable option for busy weeks.

Ingredients:

- 1 lb **boneless, skinless chicken breast**, cooked and cooled
- ⅓ cup **Butter Bacon Mayonnaise**
- 3 slices **crispy bacon**, chopped
- 1 hard-boiled **egg**, chopped *(optional)*
- **Kosher salt**, to taste

Instructions:

1. Prepare the Chicken

Dice the cooked chicken into bite-size pieces and place in a medium bowl.

2. Add Mayo & Egg

Stir in the mayonnaise and chopped egg until the chicken is fully coated and creamy.

3. Mix in Bacon

Add the chopped bacon and fold into the mixture.

4. Season and Chill

Season with salt to taste. Chill before serving for best flavor and texture.

> Serve cold with pork rinds, spooned over hard-boiled egg halves, or packed into lettuce cups for an easy meal on the go.

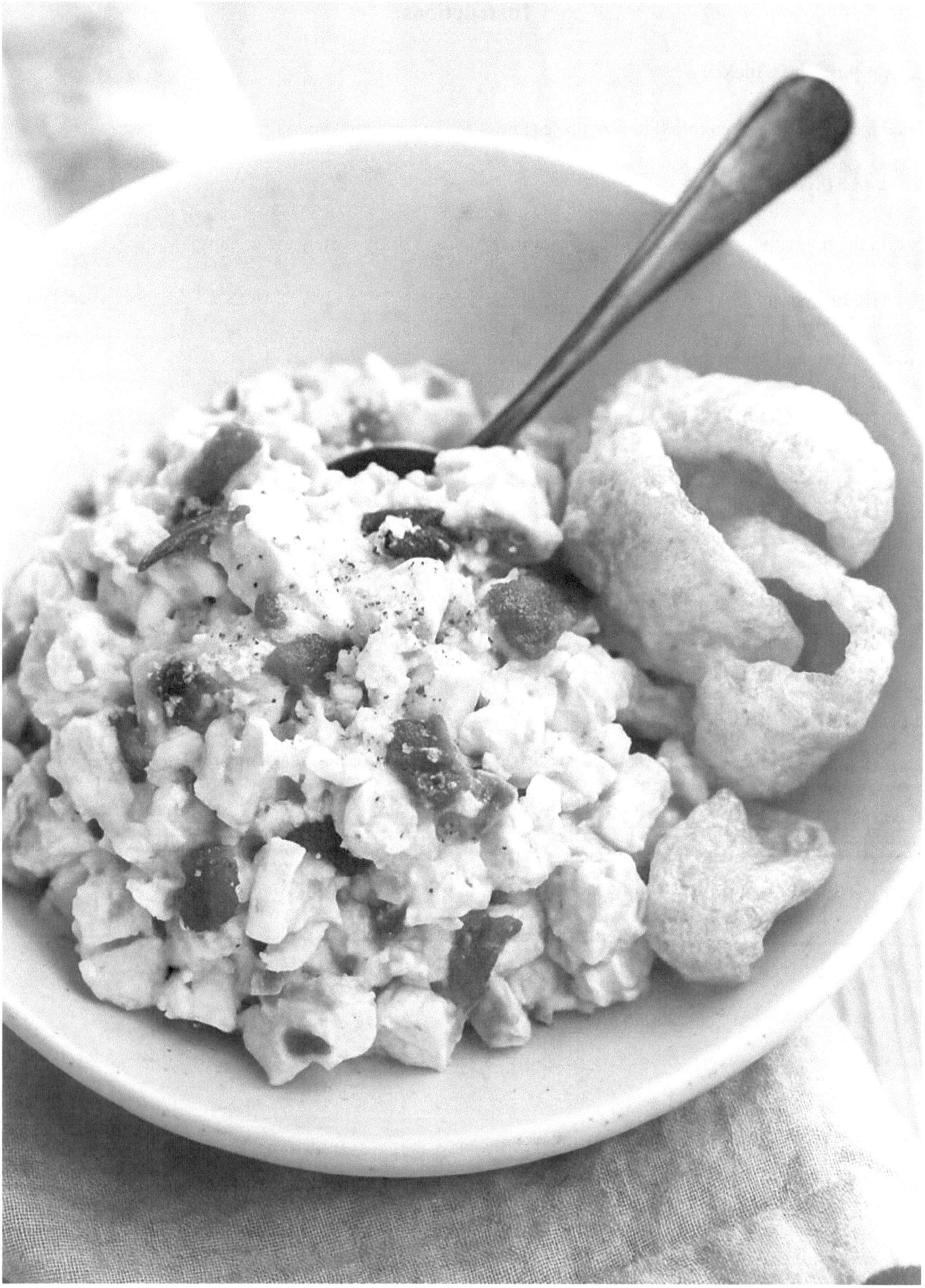

Eggs Benedict

Here's a fully carnivore-friendly take on **Eggs Benedict**—rich, indulgent, and completely free of bread, carbs, or plants. Instead of English muffins, we use seared rounds of crispy sausage or pan-fried carnivore bread. The hollandaise? Pure buttery perfection.

Carnivore Eggs Benedict

Yield: 2 servings (2 stacks)

Prep Time: 10 minutes

Cook Time: 15 minutes

Total Time: ~25 minutes

Ingredients:

Base & Toppings:

- 2 **large sausage patties** (or 2 slices of carnivore bread, toasted)
- 2 **egg yolks**
- 2 **whole eggs** (for poaching)
- 4 tbsp **unsalted butter**, melted
- 1 tsp **lemon juice** (optional, omit for strict carnivore)
- Sea salt, to taste

- Optional: 1 slice **crispy bacon** or **beef ham** per stack

Instructions:

1. **Cook the Base**

Form two thick sausage patties and pan-sear over medium heat until browned and cooked through. Set aside. (Or toast slices of carnivore bread in butter.)

2. **Poach the Eggs**

Bring water to a gentle simmer in a saucepan. Add a splash of vinegar (optional). Crack eggs into ramekins, swirl water gently, and slide eggs in. Poach for **3–4 minutes**, until whites are set. Remove with slotted spoon.

3. **Make Hollandaise**

Whisk egg yolks with a pinch of salt in a small bowl over a warm (not hot) water bath. Slowly drizzle in melted butter while whisking constantly until the sauce thickens to a silky texture. Add lemon juice if using.

4. **Assemble**

Place each sausage patty or bread slice on a plate. Top with poached egg, then spoon warm hollandaise generously over the top. Add crispy bacon or meat slices if desired.

Tips:

- For a richer version, sprinkle with crispy pork panko just before serving.
- Hollandaise can be made in a blender for speed—just pour melted butter into yolks while blending on low.

> Decadent, filling, and 100% carnivore-compliant—this Eggs Benedict hits all the right notes without a single crumb of bread.

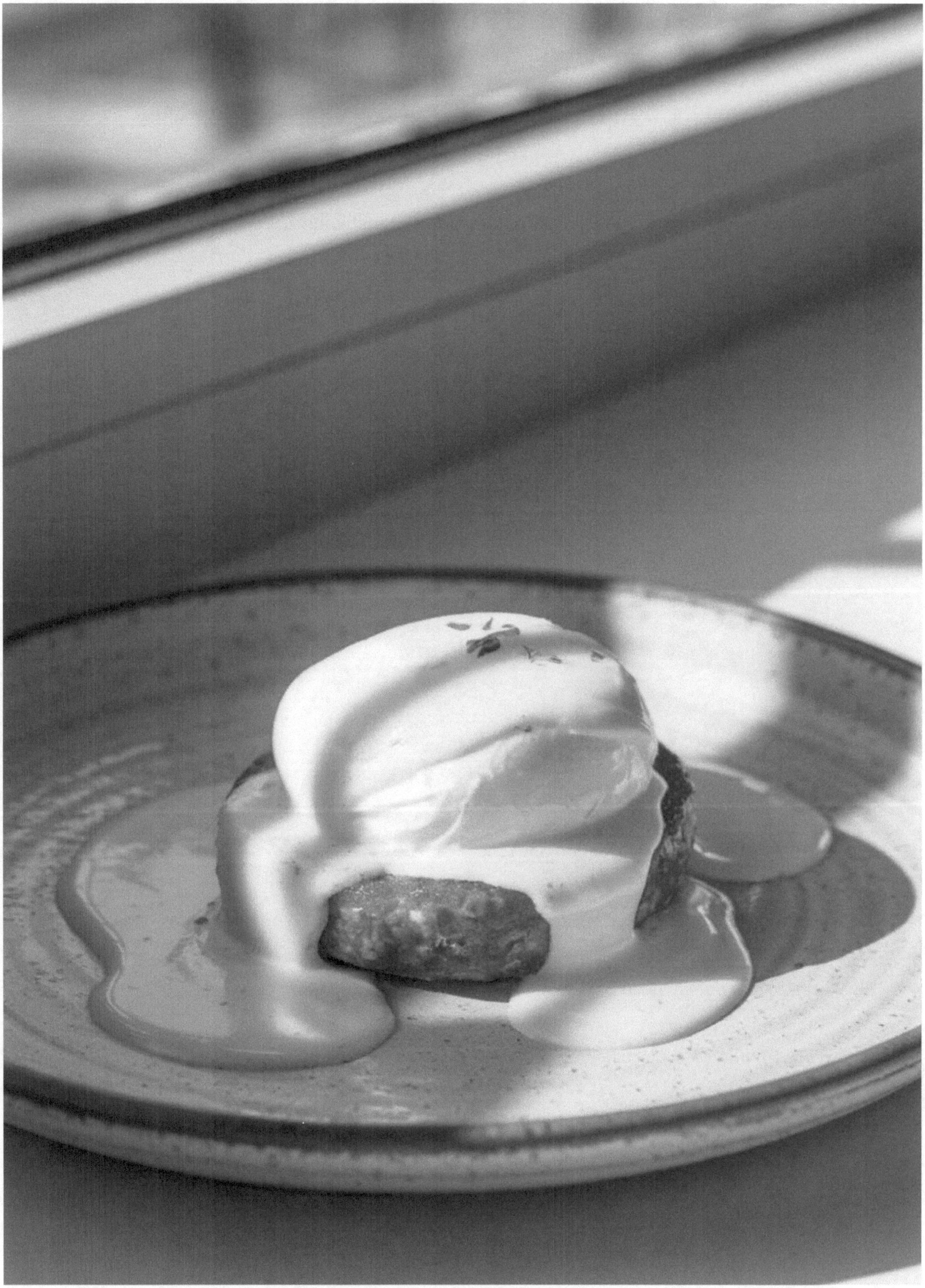

Carnivore Breakfast Burrito

Yield: 1 burrito

Prep Time: 5 minutes (not including time to cook bacon or prep tortilla)

Cook Time: 5 minutes

This hearty breakfast burrito is rich, cheesy, and ultra-satisfying—perfect for mornings when you need something portable, protein-packed, and quick. It's warm, melty, and wrapped in a low-carb, carnivore-style tortilla that doesn't skimp on flavor.

Ingredients:

- 2 **large eggs**
- 1 tbsp **heavy cream**
- 1 tbsp **butter** or **bacon grease** (for cooking)
- 1 slice **cheddar** or **gouda** cheese
- 2 slices **crispy bacon**, chopped or whole
- 1 **carnivore tortilla** (7–8 inches)
- Sea salt, to taste

Instructions:

1. **Scramble the Eggs**

In a bowl, whisk together eggs, heavy cream, and a pinch of salt. Heat butter in a skillet over medium heat, then pour in the eggs. Cook gently, stirring until soft and fluffy.

2. **Warm the Tortilla**

While eggs cook, warm your carnivore tortilla in a separate dry pan or microwave until pliable.

3. **Assemble the Burrito**

Layer the scrambled eggs onto the center of the tortilla. Top with cheese and bacon. Let the cheese melt slightly.

4. **Roll It Up**

Fold in the sides, then roll tightly from the bottom. If desired, return to the skillet seam-side down for 1–2 minutes to crisp and seal.

Tips:

- Add leftover sausage or steak strips for a meatier version.
- Store wrapped burritos in the fridge and reheat in an air fryer for on-the-go mornings.

Warm, portable, and layered with savory goodness—this is your new favorite way to eat bacon and eggs.

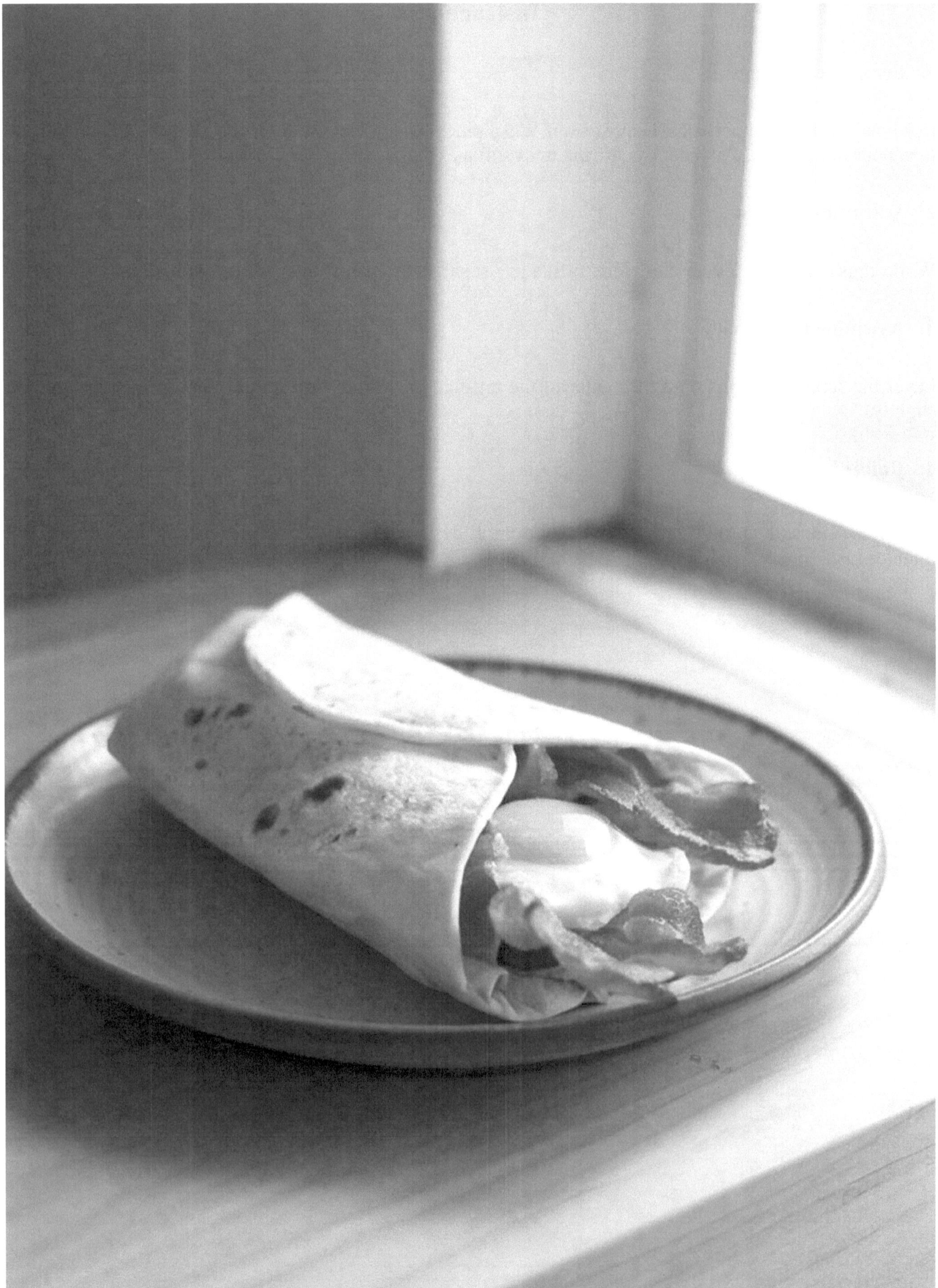

Dutch Baby Soufflé

Yield: 8 servings

Prep Time: 10 minutes

Cook Time: 30 minutes

This dish lands somewhere between a custardy pancake, a rich soufflé, and a slightly sweetened protein-packed treat. It's soft in the center, puffs dramatically in the oven, and can be served warm straight from the pan or crisped up in an air fryer for a different texture. Whether you're craving comfort food or a fun brunch dish, this one delivers.

Ingredients:

- ½ cup (1 stick) **salted butter**, melted
- ½ cup **heavy cream**
- ½ cup **unflavored, unsweetened protein powder**
- ⅓ cup **egg white powder**
- 4 **large eggs**
- 1 (8-ounce) package **cream cheese**, softened
- 1 tbsp **unflavored powdered gelatin**
- ¼ tsp **kosher salt**
- 1 tsp **vanilla extract**
- 1½ tsp **ground cinnamon**, divided

Instructions:

1. Preheat the Oven

Preheat to **375°F (190°C)**. Line an **8-inch square baking pan** with parchment paper, covering the bottom and sides.

2. Blend the Batter

In a food processor or high-speed blender, combine all ingredients except ½ tsp of the cinnamon. Blend until smooth and creamy. Pour into the prepared pan.

3. Add Cinnamon Swirl

Sprinkle the remaining cinnamon evenly over the top and swirl with a toothpick or the tip of a knife to create a light marbled effect.

4. Bake

Bake for **30 minutes**, or until puffed, golden brown on top, and set in the center. A toothpick should come out clean when inserted into the middle.

5. Serve

Let cool slightly (it will deflate—don't worry). Slice into 8 pieces. Serve warm, or reheat slices in an air fryer at 400°F for 3–5 minutes until crispy and golden on the edges.

Serving Suggestions:

- Top with whipped butter or drizzle with melted tallow or cream.
- Store leftovers in the fridge and crisp them up for a satisfying snack or breakfast later.

> Puffy, soft, and lightly spiced—this soufflé is as fun to make as it is to eat.

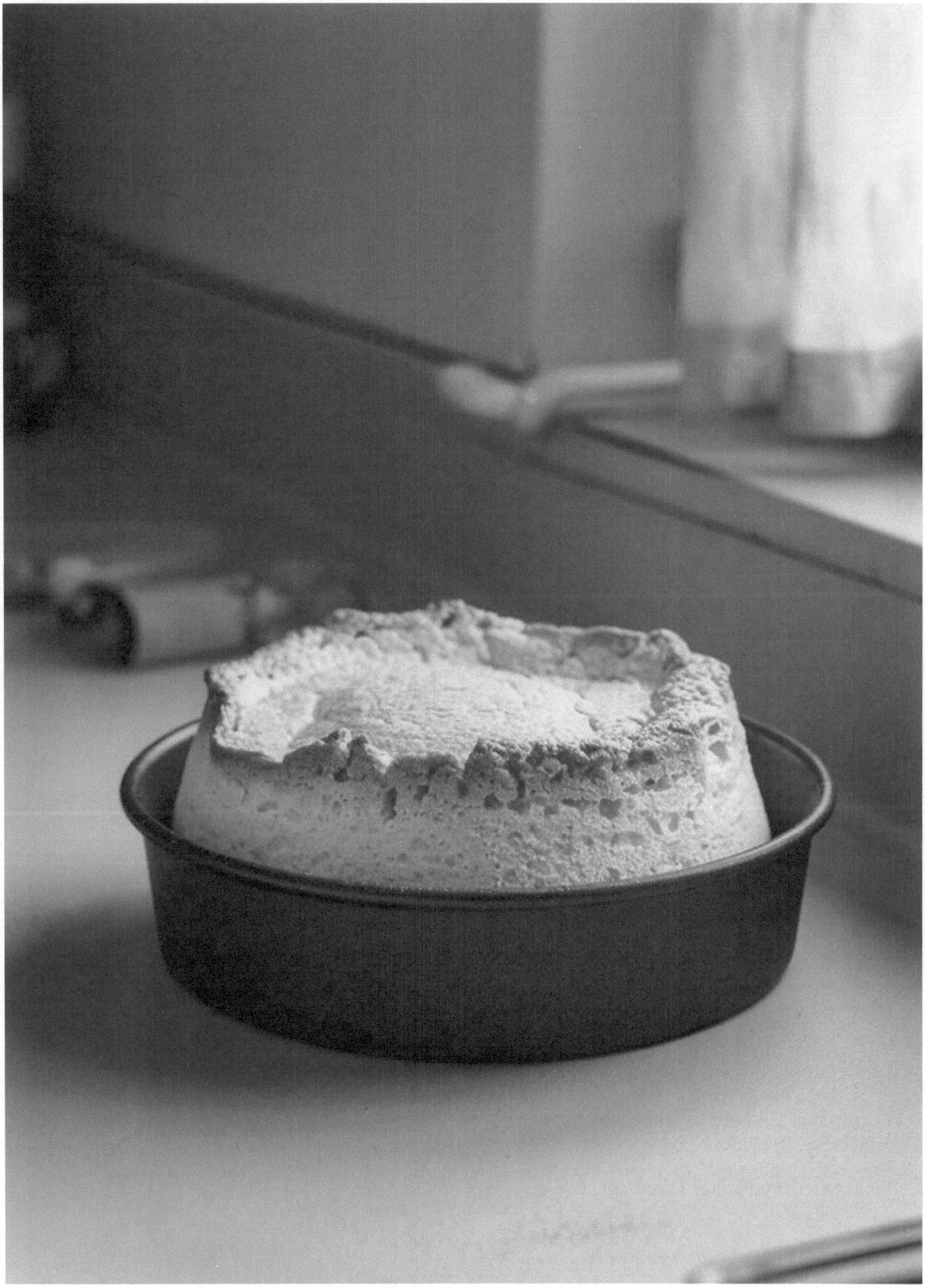

Carnivore Ice Cream — 3 Ways

Yield: 2 servings

Prep Time: 5 minutes, plus time to churn

Rich, creamy, and totally indulgent—this carnivore-style ice cream hits the sweet spot without any sugar, carbs, or plants (unless you choose to go wild with add-ins). Whether you're in the mood for something simple like vanilla, bold like coffee, or decadent like cheesecake, the base is easy to customize. Perfect for celebrations, lazy weekends, or anytime you want to enjoy a frozen treat that fits your lifestyle.

For the Base:

- 1 cup **heavy cream**
- 2 large **egg yolks**

Flavor Options:

Vanilla Ice Cream (Makes 1½ cups):

- 1 teaspoon **vanilla extract**
- Tiny pinch **sea salt**
- Optional: ½ teaspoon **cream cheese** for extra creaminess

Coffee Ice Cream (Makes 1½ cups):

- 1 teaspoon **instant espresso powder**

- Tiny pinch **salt**
- Optional: ½ teaspoon **butter** for richness

Cheesecake Ice Cream (Makes 2 cups):

- 3 oz (6 tbsp) **cream cheese**
- ½ teaspoon **vanilla extract**
- 1 tablespoon **whipped butter** or ghee (optional for a smoother finish)

For Serving:

- Freshly whipped cream (unsweetened)

Special Equipment:

- Ice cream maker

Instructions:

1. Blend

Add the base ingredients plus your chosen flavor ingredients to a blender. Blend until completely smooth. If using cream cheese, ensure there are no lumps.

2. Churn

Pour into your ice cream maker and churn according to the manufacturer's instructions (typically 10–15 minutes). The texture should resemble soft-serve.

3. Freeze (Optional)

Enjoy immediately or transfer to the freezer to firm up for a more scoopable consistency.

4. Serve

Top with whipped cream and enjoy! If frozen solid, let it sit at room temperature for a few minutes before scooping.

Tips:

- For a smoother texture, add a touch of butter or ghee while blending.
- Store leftovers in an airtight container and enjoy within 30 days for best flavor

> This creamy treat is endlessly adaptable, deeply satisfying, and proof that carnivore life doesn’t mean skipping dessert.

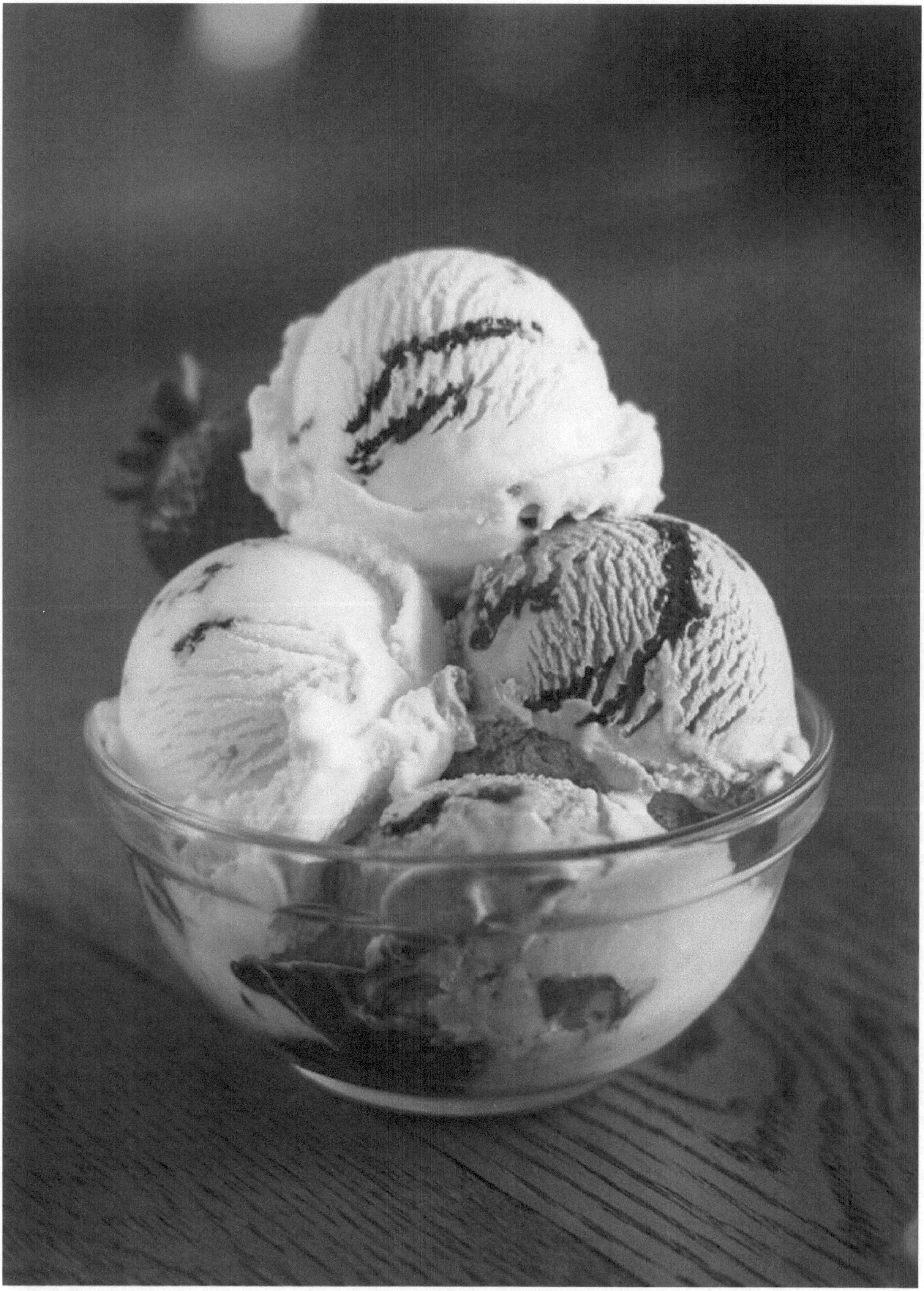

Ice Cream Sandwiches

Yield: 6 servings

Prep Time: 25 minutes, plus chill time (not including time to make ice cream)

Cook Time: 15 minutes

What started as a humble cookie evolved into the ultimate frozen treat. These ice cream sandwiches are rich, creamy, and easy to store for grab-and-go indulgence. Keep a batch in the freezer—you'll be glad you did.

For the Cookies:

- ¼ cup (½ stick) **salted butter**, softened
- 3 **large egg yolks**
- 1 **large whole egg**
- 2 tsp **vanilla extract**
- 1 tbsp **cream cheese**, softened
- ¼ cup **collagen powder**
- 1¼ cups (115 g) **pork panko**
- 1½ tsp **ground cinnamon**

Filling:

- Double batch **Vanilla Ice Cream** (see note)

Instructions:

1. In a medium bowl, beat the butter, egg yolks, whole egg, vanilla, and cream cheese with a hand mixer on medium speed until smooth and creamy.
2. Add the collagen and mix until fully blended. Stir in pork panko and cinnamon until a sticky dough forms.
3. Freeze the dough for 15 minutes or until it firms up enough to handle easily.
4. While the dough chills, preheat oven to **400°F (200°C)** and line a baking sheet with parchment.
5. Divide the dough into 12 equal portions. Roll each into a ball, place on the sheet, and press into thin, ¼-inch rounds, about 3 inches wide.
6. Bake for 15 minutes, or until edges are golden. Let cool on the pan a few minutes to reabsorb some of the melted fat.
7. Transfer cookies to a wire rack. Let cool completely while softening the ice cream slightly on the counter.
8. Spread about ½ cup of softened ice cream onto one cookie, then top with a second cookie. Repeat to make six sandwiches.
9. Wrap each sandwich tightly in plastic wrap and freeze until firm, at least 2 hours.
10. Let sit at room temperature for a few minutes before eating if very firm. Store leftovers in the freezer for up to a month.

Blue Cheese Cream Sauce

Yield: About 1 cup (4 to 6 servings)

Prep Time: 5 minutes

Cook Time: 5 minutes

This rich and velvety sauce is perfect drizzled over steaks, burgers, or even mixed into shredded beef or pork. It's equally good served warm or chilled, with its flavor deepening as it rests. Keep extra on hand—you'll want to spoon it on everything.

Ingredients:

- ½ cup **heavy cream**
- 1 tbsp **unsalted butter**
- 1 cup **crumbled blue cheese** (about 4 ounces), plus extra for garnish

Instructions:

1. In a small saucepan over medium-low heat, combine the cream and butter. Heat gently until the butter melts and the mixture starts to steam.
2. Stir in the blue cheese and whisk occasionally until the cheese is mostly melted and the sauce is smooth and slightly thickened, about 5 minutes.
3. Serve warm, or chill for a thicker texture. Garnish with extra crumbled blue cheese if desired.

Serving Suggestions:

- Spoon over grilled steak, pan-seared chicken thighs, or crispy pork belly.
- Use as a dip for cold roast beef slices or meatballs.
- Store in an airtight container in the fridge for up to 4 days; reheat gently to serve again.

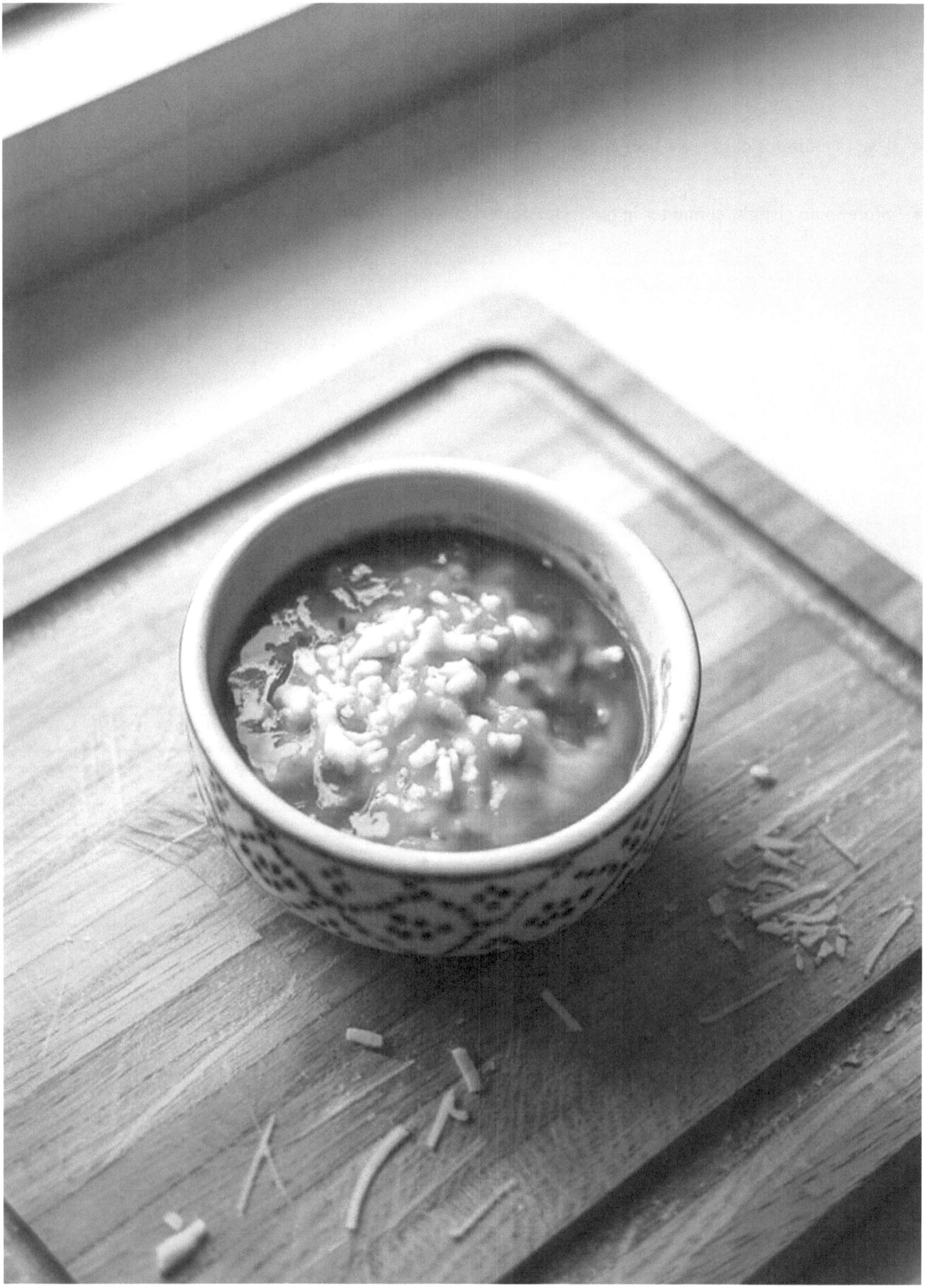